Publisher's Note: This is a work of fiction. Names, characters, places, and incidents are a product of the author's imagination. Locales and public names are sometimes used for atmospheric purposes. Any resemblance to actual people, living or dead, or to businesses, companies, events, institutions, or locales is completely coincidental.

This book is not intended as a substitute for the medical advice of physicians. The reader should regularly consult a physician in matters relating to his/her health and particularly with respect to any symptoms that may require diagnosis or medical attention. (*health, alternative healing*) Before beginning any new exercise program it is recommended that you seek medical advice from your personal physician.

#Workoutkingboxset

http://workoutkingrule.blogspot.com/

workoutkingrule@gmail.com

<u>The Workout King Box Set</u>

The Sprint Diet

The Jump Rope Diet

The Kettlebell Cleanse

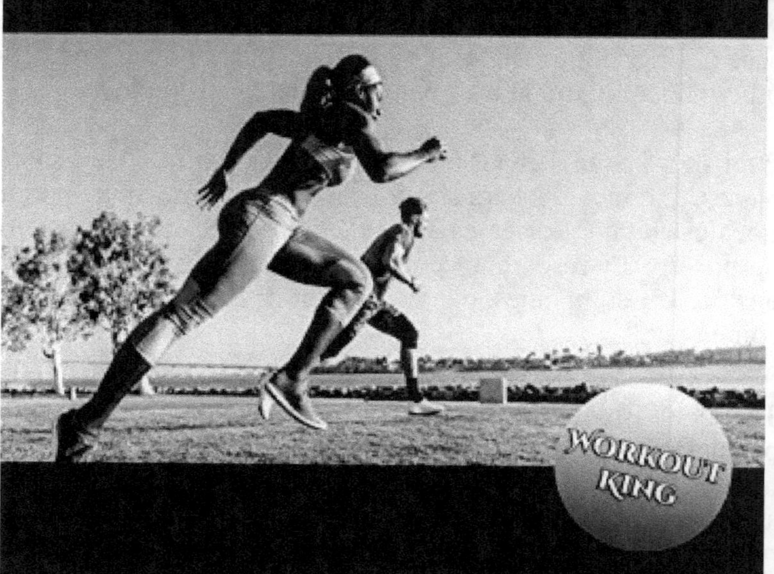

WORKOUT KING
THE SPRINT DIET
3 MIN WEIGHT LOSS HIIT TRAINING

The Sprint Diet

My Story

If you're looking for someone that's going to use fancy words and bullshit to sell you on a good comprehensive workout than you've come to the wrong place. If you're looking for someone who's going to use periods and commas in the right place than you've come to the wrong place. This is going to be straightforward and to the point. I'm not going to sit here and bullshit you. I'm not going to give you information that didn't work for me because that would be stupid and completely misleading.

Let me tell you my story. I was a regular attractive young guy and then I got in a relationship. Once that happened I gain an extremely large amount of weight. The next thing you know I'm not in a relationship anymore and I'm 50 pounds heavier. I've never had to lose weight a day in my life. I've never had to watch my calories. I've never had to exercise. All this shit was completely new to me. If I had a time machine I would go back and say hey dumbass just sprint.

       Sprinting makes perfect sense it's the most effective workout in the world and it only takes you a couple of minutes. Sprinting just makes common sense. I tried every single one of those machines in the gym. I tried the elliptical the bike and of course the fucking treadmill. Now for anybody who's been in the gym for longer than ah month you've seen people use these machines. Ask yourself do they look any different? Has anything changed about them whatsoever? Most likely not! That's not to say those machines don't work but if your goal is to lose weight than those machines are not the answer. They say if you want to lose weight the best way to do it is to diet. If you workout for about a month you may have lost about 10 pounds on the treadmill but gained 10 pounds of muscle so when you get on the scale you're going to weigh the same. Most people don't understand that your body is composed of muscle and fat so they're going to think they didn't lose any weight. Most likely they're going to give up because they think working out isn't effective. I've given up many of times and I have the stretch marks to prove it but once I discovered sprinting I started to understand how the body works. You might be an individual who is composed of 50% body fat and 50% muscle. That's not good! That means you're extremely overweight. For men anything above 30% is high body fat. 21-30% is excess fat. 13-20% is moderately lean. 9-12% body fat is lean. 5-8% body fat is ultra lean but anything below 5% is risky because you have to have some fat to protect internal organs, provide energy, and regulate hormones. For women it's different. Anything above 40% is risky high body fat. 31-40% is excess fat. 23-30% is moderately lean. 19-22% body fat is lean. 15-18% is ultra lean and anything below 15% is risky low body fat.

If you want to change your body fat you have to increase the amount of muscle you have in your body. When you increase the amount of muscle you have in your body you burn fat more efficiently therefore making your day even more effective. You want to increase the amount of calories you burn at rest. That means you want to increase the amount of calories you burn doing absolutely nothing but sitting on your ass. This is called the resting metabolic rate. Your resting metabolic rate is highly affected by your muscle and your mitochondria. So what increases the amount of muscle that you have and increases the amount of mitochondria you have? If your answer is sprinting you're correct! As a matter of fact sprinting is the only exercise that can burn fat and build muscle at the same time. I realized that the three hours I was spending on the elliptical was a complete and utter waste of time I could literally get the same results by sprinting for 3 minutes.

The Benefits Of Sprinting

Sprinting will help you build strength and power in your fast-twitch fibers. Fast twitch fibers are what you use when you punch as fast and as hard as you can. You use your fast twitch fibers when you exert yourself as hard as you possibly can in any exercise. It's basically the number one muscle that you would use in a flight or fight situation. Sprinting also increases protein synthesis pathways by as much as 230% helping you build stronger muscles faster. Protein synthesis is probably one of the most important factors to building muscle.

When you're on a treadmill or ah elliptical you have absolutely no idea what it is that your body is burning. You could be burning muscle. You could be burning sugar. You could be burning carbohydrates. When you're sprinting you're definitely burning fat sprinting isn't going to change the number on the scale but it is going to change the number on your measuring tape. You lose body fat not body mass that's because your body more effectively burns fat when it's exerting its self at a higher intensity. To put it is numbers your body burns fat better when you're giving your workout 47 to 64% effort. Basically the more intense the workout is the more likely it is that you're burning fat. Less intensity increases the likelihood of you burning various other fuel sources in your body. So if you're a person with a lot of fat on your body that's the most dominant fuel source available so when you're exerting yourself at a high intensity of course your body is going to reach for it's most dominant fuel source.

Sprinting literally trains the body to burn fat for fuel so you can preserve muscle glycogen and prolong your workout. This is why it increases your endurance so significantly. If you are a long distance runner you want to sprint to increase your energy and endurance. By going at max speed you amplify your oxygen uptake and when you do that you increase the time it takes for fatigue to set in. To put it simple you increase the amount of mitochondria in your body and mitochondria is responsible for energy production. Mitochondria takes fat, sugar, muscle, carbohydrates, and other resources in your body and converts them into ATP. ATP is the energy currency of your body so the more mitochondria you have the more efficient your body is at creating energy. The more efficient your body is at creating energy the longer you can run, the longer you can jump, and the longer you can lift.

Sprinting also increases the speed and power of an individual because it's essentially speed training. Sprinting is exactly what a track star does to train. Track stars sprint to increase the strength of their fast twitch muscles, which are responsible for their speed. So the more you sprint the faster you become. Sprinting also lowers blood pressure because it increases the power of your fast-twitch muscles, which improve heart function significantly. Exerting that explosive energy will make your heart pump harder which will strengthen it and decrease the likelihood of you contracting a heart disease. Sprinting saves time because you only need to do 2 minutes and 30 seconds of it a day to receive the same results that you would get from about an hour to 30 minutes of aerobic exercise. It also builds mental toughness as well because they're going to be times that you want to give up. Overcoming this feeling will strengthen your resolve.

Sprinting is probably the hardest form of exercise that you possibly can do because it's the most demanding form of exercise there is. Still since you don't have to do very much of it sprinting has the benefit of saving you a significant amount of time. You don't have to worry about working it around your work schedule. It won't get in the way of you taking care of your children. You don't need to call a baby sitter. It literally is something you can do right before you go to bed or right when you wake up in the morning.

For 2 minutes and 30 seconds of exercise a day you can reduce your stress. When you sprint you produce a significant amount of endorphins, which are like your body's natural painkillers. You'll get a strong euphoric sensation from this type of exercise. The best way to describe it is to call it what it is, it's a high probably one of the best highs you can get without using a substance. Sprinting improves glucose control, which helps you regulate your insulin so that you don't get high cholesterol, high blood pressure, or high blood sugar, and of course abdominal body fat. It does this because it completely drains the body of glycogen, which than releases the sugar stored inside of our muscles.

Now for the Holy Grail of sprinting, it is the most effective exercise on abdominal belly fat! Number one it makes your abdominals contract more than any other exercise. Number two it improves glucose control, which is a major cause of abdominal body fat. To put it simple sprinting helps you burn fat and prevent new fat from forming. Sprinting increases your energy level and your endurance. By increasing energy and endurance you can work out longer and harder. By increasing mitochondria you also increase your metabolic rate, which means you burn more fat at rest. It's literally the most effective exercise you could possibly do and it doesn't take you any time to do at all.

So why is no one sprinting? Most people don't even know about it, it's not the most famous form of exercise. Unlike the elliptical, stair climber, treadmill, and bike sprinting doesn't really have a big voice. Athletes are the exception because they understand the benefits of sprinting. This is why they're in better physical shape than everyone else on the planet. Sprinting is why Usain Bolt is the fastest man in the world. It's why all your favorite basketball players are able to play non-stop without passing out. It's why long distance runners continue to set records. It's the one exercise that takes you from being fit to being an athlete to being an Olympian.

Beginners Guide

Now this is where plenty of mistakes are made. When you first start sprinting you don't want to over exert yourself. The best method is to do six ten second sprints that one minute. Make sure you go full out I mean no holds bars. If you sit down after the sprint and you still have energy left than you didn't sprint. Sprinting should leave you absolutely exhausted. There shouldn't be anything left in the tank. If there is than you need to sprint harder. You might need to increase the amount of time that you sprint. If you still have energy after ten seconds I would suggest four fifteen-second sprints. By sprinting for a minute every single day you'll start to notice the changes in your body. Your energy will start increasing and your stress will go down.

Before I go on any longer I probably should explain the stress that sprinting can have on your joints. This is why you should never sprint on cement. Even Olympic sprinters don't run on cement. To be honest they don't train on the track every single day because the track is an incredibly hard surface. Most sprinters run on grass or dirt. The smartest thing you could do is run on sand it's a very difficult surface to move on and the added drag makes the sprint that much more effective not to mention the surface isn't aggressive on your joints at all. Me personally I sprint on carpet usually I'll get a yoga mat and place it on top of my carpet than I'll sprint in place. Sprinting in place is very effective to be honest it's just as effective as a moving sprint. As long as you exert yourself to complete exhaustion you're on the right track.

Let me explain my process in better detail. You can either do it my way or you can find your own way of doing it. Just make sure the surface you're sprinting on is soft. First I lay my yoga mat down on the floor and fold it in half. Second I turn my fan on and face it towards my resting place so basically the spot I'm going to sit after I do my sprint. I place my water bottle right next to my rest area because you have to remain hydrated especially when you're exerting this amount of energy. If you don't stay hydrated it could be dangerous. I take my computer out and go to Google. I type in timer. Google has a timer app that appears in the search engine. You can either set ah alarm or you can use the stopwatch feature. For this exercise I use the stopwatch feature. When I'm ready I press start and than I immediately start pumping my arms and legs as fast as I possibly can. I don't lift my knees up super high because that lowers your speed a lot. I want to move my legs as fast as I can so keeping my knees below my waist is important. I make sure to keep up right so that my core is stabilized. By keeping upright I make sure that I get the maximum abdominal benefit from the exercise. If you lean forward too much your core isn't holding up your upper body, which means it's not being properly worked out. Make sure you run on the balls of your feet not your heels. Now staying in the same spot isn't something I'm very good at. I usually end up all over the room. You want to stabilize your position so that you stay in the same spot especially because you don't want to move off the yoga mat. At no point do you want to decrease your speed you have to be at full intensity for the entire 10-second duration of the sprint otherwise it's not a sprint. Once I see the stopwatch reach 10 seconds I immediately sit down. Never count out the seconds you'll get it wrong ever time use some sort of stopwatch.

The breeze of the fan helps me to relax and recover as I drink some water. Since you're new to this exercise you want to rest until you're ready for the next run. You don't want to put a time limit on your rest. Once you become more acquainted with ten second sprints you want to keep your rest periods down to about 30 seconds unless your doing 30 second sprints than your going to need two minutes of rest. In the beginning you might rest from 1 minute to 2 minutes or even 5 minutes in between each sprint. Now when I'm done with my 6th sprint I'm usually completely wiped out I try to recover by drinking plenty of water and resting until I'm ready to move again. The feeling that I have after my 6th sprint is a combination of fatigue and euphoria. It's a weird kind of high that I can't really explain but the more you sprint the better the high gets. Now you want to do these one-minute sprints everyday for at least 1 week than you want to try to add more sprints to your regiment. The beginning goal is to go from 6 to 12 ten second sprints so you're doing a total of 2 minutes of sprints everyday. Your secondary goal is to go from 12 ten-second sprints to eight 15 second sprints, which is still two minutes but you've increased how long you can run per sprint which is incredibly important. You can stretch before and after you do this sprinting routine. I personally don't that's probably because I sprint in place I don't sprint on a track or outdoors so there isn't too much impact on my joints. For me sprinting in place is much more demanding than an actual moving sprint probably because I can move my body faster when I'm sprinting in place compared to a moving sprint.

You want to make sure you move your arms back and forth from about your ear to your hip. The faster you pump your arms the faster your body will move. When I first started sprinting after about the third day pretty much all the muscles in my body became sore I had to take about two to three days off and than start sprinting again but after that I never became sore again. That happened because the various muscles that I was using to conduct the sprint hadn't been used through all of my other workouts especially not at that intensity. I had extreme muscle soreness in my back which was surprising to me at first until I took into account the intensity in which I was swinging my arms they were going all the way back than all the way forward so I was activating muscles in my back that I had never activated before. If this beginner s*** is to easy for you start off at an intermediate lever. If that's easy for you start off at ah advance level.

Intermediate Guide

Once you can do eight 15-second sprints than you've reached the intermediate level. Now when most people reach this level they always want to start using different devices when they sprint. People want to get on the treadmill and sprint, which by the way is horrible for your joints especially for your knees. Do not sprint on the treadmill! Sprinting on the treadmill is incredibly dangerous! You never want to sprint on a hard moving surface nothing about that sounds like a good idea. Make sure you stay away from surfaces that can be strenuous on your joints. Some individuals want to sprint on bikes this I would recommend because there's virtually no impact whatsoever. The only difference from sprinting on a bike and sprinting in place is that there's no arm movement so you might be able to sprint on a bike longer than you would be able to sprint in place. Some individuals want to sprint using the elliptical. Elliptical sprinting is not intermediate sprinting you're not ready to sprint on an elliptical yet.

If you are on an intermediate level you have just a few goals. The first goal is to go from eight 15-second sprints to six 20-second sprints. So you'll still be doing two-minute sprints you'll just be increasing the duration of each individual sprint. Once you get to this point you want to hold it here for about a week. After a week you want to add another sprint to the equation so you're doing 7 twenty-second sprints. The next week you want to do eight. The week after that you want to do 9. Once you reach nine 20 second sprints you've reached the advanced level. Now don't worry if you're not capable of following this week by week plan go at your own pace. As long as you wind up doing 9 twenty second sprints you'll be okay. Take your time and give your body rest. Once you're doing nine 20 second sprints you're doing 3 minutes of sprinting every single day that's advanced level s*** right there. Give yourself a huge pat on the back for having that much power because that's what sprint accomplishments are advancement in power. Your body is literally becoming more powerful every single day because you're increasing the amount of mitochondria in your body, which means your energy levels are going up every single day.

Advance Sprinting

Now there are many goals once you get to advanced sprinting. First and foremost you want to go from nine 20-second sprints to six 30-second sprints. You'll still be doing 3 minutes of sprinting but you'll be increasing your time per sprint. Now this might be the last time you increase your time per sprint. 30 seconds to me should be the max. Some people can do 60 seconds sprints if you can reach that point than by all means go there. 60-second sprints would be a 400-meter dash. 30-second sprints would be 250-meter dash. 20-second sprints would be a 200-meter dash. 10-second sprints would be a 100-meter dash. If 30 seconds becomes easy than increase your time to 35, 40, 45, 50, 55, and than 60. Just three sixty-second sprints is murder but you could max out at 6 sixty-second sprints. Mind you that is insanity six 30-second all out sprints is plenty especially if you're sprinting in place because you don't have to lift your knees up incredibly high. Lifting your knees up incredibly high reduces your speed so of course you're sprint will last longer. Now the last thing you want to do is add one more 30-second sprint to your regiment maxing you out at 3 minutes and 30 seconds. That's seven 30-second sprints. Once you reach this point you're truly ready for some advanced level sprinting.

You're probably reading this and thinking that this sounds crazy because 3 minutes and 30 seconds of exercise doesn't sound like a long time but once you actually start sprinting you'll look at this section differently. To be honest once you start sprinting this might even seem impossible. Having this level of energy will make you feel like you're 15 again, which makes sense because mitochondria is directly related to aging.

Mitochondria are an entirely separate organism they has their own DNA our relationship with them begin a long, long, long, time ago. Do to free radicals the communication between our two genomes brakes down over time causing major problems. The best way to prevent this from happening is to sprint. Sprinting is the most effective way to increase the body's mitochondrial function keeping you energetic young and healthy.

Now that you've reached a truly advanced level with sprinting you can start to add some extra spice to your workout the first thing I would recommend trying is leg weights. Leg weights are incredibly effective at increasing the difficulty of your sprint workout. I would recommend that you do not go over 5 pounds on each leg. Once you go over 5 pounds on each leg you risk injury because the heavier the leg weights are the more they move around. I usually put 2.5 pounds on each leg it's a lot easier to manage and I don't have to worry about the leg weights moving around. Even five pounds on each leg can be tricky if you don't have the right kind of leg weights. The increased resistance really makes the workout much more rewarding. Most people are not able to adjust to having leg weights on because it creates an imbalance between the arms and the legs if this is the case than you want to wear arm weights as well. Make sure that they are the exact weight otherwise you'll throw off your equilibrium. So 2.5 pounds on each leg and 2.5 pounds on each arm adding a total of 10 pounds to your body.

Now if you're doing moving sprints than a weight vest would be effective but if you were sprinting in place a weighted vest wouldn't be very effective. Sprinting on sand is incredibly effective it's probably one of the most difficult sprint workouts you can do and adding leg weights, arm weights, and ah weighted vests would make it even more difficult. That's real advanced sprint training. Hill sprints are a favorite amongst athletes just make sure the hill you're running up isn't concrete. Run up a grass hill or a dirt hill.

Now all these things are fine and all but the most advanced form of sprint training in my opinion is elliptical sprint training. Not only is it the most advanced form of sprint training but it's also the safest form of sprint training because it's virtually zero impact. Elliptical sprinting is resistance sprinting. You can continue to increase the resistance on the machine making it more and more difficult for you to sprint making the workout that much more effective. You want to turn the resistance up until it's actually difficult for you to move than you sprint your ass off. You want it to be so difficult that you can only sprint for 10 seconds. You want to do 6 ten second sprints. You want to continue doing this until this resistance level becomes easy for you. Than you want to increase your time following the beginner, intermediate, and advance formula all over again. This kind of workout was literally a life-changer for me. I went from 250 pounds 50% body fat to

200 pounds 13% body fat and all I did was work out for 3 minutes and 30 seconds a day.

It's very important to know what your body is made of. You want to measure your resting metabolic rate and you're fat and muscle content. The best way to do that is to use the bod pod. Look up the bod pod online and find out if one is near you. Your gym might already have one it might cost you anywhere from $40 to $60 to use it but it's incredibly worth it. It's like getting a detailed diagnostic on your bodies composition. Actually it is getting a detailed diagnostic of your body's composition.

The Kettlebell Cleanse

Sprinting is incredibly powerful still if you combine it with weight training it becomes that much more powerful. Now most people don't have time to go to the gym to use complex weight training equipment that's why the best solution is to use the Kettlebell. The Kettlebell is a tested and proven tool not to mention it's one of the only forms of weight training that burns and extremely large amount of calories. 3 hours of kettlebell training would burn 3600 calories that's a pound + 100 calories. The kettlebell works out every single inch of the body so you don't have to worry about getting any other machine. It can do everything that all the complex machines in the gym can do and it's only one tool. You just have to make sure that the weight is difficult if the weight is not at least slightly difficult than you're wasting your time. With 15 minutes of kettlebell training plus obeying the sprint diet you can lose a significant amount of weight fast. To learn more about kettlebell training check out my other book "The Kettlebell Cleanse" coming soon.

What's Your Motivation

Now I'm not going to lie to you this type of exercise is incredibly difficult. It's quick and to the point but it's difficult. A lot of people are going to give up because this s*** is probably the hardest form of exercise that your ever going to do. The number one benefit is it's not time consuming. The number two benefit is it's incredibly effective it's the most effective form of exercise on the planet. Nothing will challenge your body more. Nothing will sculpt your body more. Nothing will change your internal chemistry more. This is what makes it the best exercise in the world. Once you start doing it you won't want to stop. It'll become like a drug trust me I'm addicted to this shit. Still getting started will be difficult because your body won't be use to exerting so much energy. The amount of stress that it puts on your energy reserves is amazing but that's what makes you stronger and more energetic. You have to destroy your body so that it can rebuild itself stronger and better. Your body likes to adapt as quickly as it possibly can. This is why exercise eventually becomes easy to you. Your body will adapt to the different complex movements that are involved in aerobic exercise and some forms of weight lifting as well. The only exercise that your body can't get use to is sprinting because it's the one exercise that completely over taxes the body. That means as long as you sprint there will always be progression. All you have to do is add more time but only seconds not hours. Still even knowing this when you actually get up and do it your going to realize what I'm talking about this s*** is no walk in the park. This is for people that are serious about changing their health. Overall aerobic exercise like the treadmill, the elliptical, or the bike will definitely help you in the long run but sprinting changes your health on another level it extends your life without taking away so much of it. Other exercises are literally going to add up to days and months of your life because they're time-consuming there's hours involved. When you look back over your life you're going to realize that a large majority of it was spent just working out when really all you needed was two minutes and 30 seconds. Three minutes and 30 seconds if you're a pro.

You need to find your motivation right now! Did you recently get dumped and you want to create that revenge body that says hey you f***** up? Did you recently get diagnosed with high blood pressure and you want to make sure that you're here to see another day? Did you recently get diagnosed with diabetes and you want to make sure your family doesn't have to bury you before your time? Do you have absolutely no energy whatsoever and it's making your life a living hell? Or do you just want to be sexy as f***? No matter which one of these things applies to you sprinting will help you with it. More energy, better health, better sex, and better looks you can't beat that. Not to mention enhanced strength, speed, and focus. You might as well call this s*** the Superman workout. Just remember whatever your motivation is let that s*** sink down deep within you don't let it go. Let it guide you let it take over you because if you reach the point where it becomes too difficult and you say it's not worth it you'll realize your motivation wasn't strong enough. You need to be motivated you need to be consumed by your reasoning for this otherwise you will give up.

      One thing that I love about the Sprint Diet is you can look down on all the other bullshit workouts that your friends are doing. You can look down on all the bullshit you see people in the gym doing because once you start doing this you'll realize that shit is easy. You'll start to see yourself as a real athlete and start looking at those other guys in the gym as lite weights. What they're doing isn't nearly as hard as this. That sense of pride will guide you and push you even further it'll make you feel like you're the s*** and sometimes that's all we need. Sometimes the best motivation on the planet is feeling like you're the s***. My motivation was pretty much every fucking thing on that list. I had high blood pressure. I was pre-diabetic. I had just got dumped and I wanted to be sexy as f***. Those things were ingrained in me. That's all I could think about every single day. I was fixated on it to the point where it became an extreme obsession. The obsessive nature of my thinking was the source of my motivation it pushed me forward every single day. I didn't want high blood pressure because I wanted to make sure that I stayed around to see how the world unfolded. I definitely didn't want diabetes because my grandma died of diabetes and watching her go through that was one of the most excruciating things I've ever dealt with. I had absolutely no energy whatsoever. I could barely stand up without feeling tired. I was always tired. I was always cranky. I was always annoyed with everything. That's how you feel when you have no energy. You feel like everything sucks. You don't want to go anywhere. You don't want to do anything. You don't want to see anyone. You just want to rest. Still no matter how much you rest you still feel tired. It was a horrible experience! Most of all I just wanted to be sexy as f*** I know that sounds a little shallow but at the end of the day we all want to be sexy. We don't want to admit it to anyone else s*** we don't even want to admit it to ourselves. Everyone wants to be sexy, beautiful, attractive whatever the hell you want to call it you want it and you can have it for the low price of 2 minutes and 30 seconds of hard work.

Vitamin Intake

Let me start this off by saying that by no means am I telling you to buy any of these vitamins I'm just telling you the vitamins that I used during the Sprint Diet. I have no idea if they had an effect on my results but I feel like they're worth mentioning. My vitamin intake during the Sprint Diet was well rounded. I tried to make sure I covered every single function of my body. Let's start things off with the first vitamin I took.

Ubiquinol is said to be very good for your cardiovascular health and the last thing I wanted going out on me was my heart because I had high blood pressure. Ubiquinol was a supplement I took to make sure I had a little extra energy. Its supposed to be an incredibly powerful antioxidant it's also supposed to promote energy production as well and I needed all the energy that I could get. They say it's good for brain health and protecting the cells from free radicals. To be honest I still use ubiquinol it's much better than Co q-10 because it's easily absorb into the body.

The second thing I kind of supplemented with was apple cider vinegar with mother. I mixed my apple cider vinegar with a teaspoon of lemon juice, eight ounces of water, and made sure to take this every single day at least 2 times a day. I have no idea what kind of effect it may have had on my progression. I just know that it's still apart of my routine to this day. Apple cider vinegar is supposed to promote weight loss. I have no idea if it contributed to my weight loss but I feel like it's worth mentioning.

The third supplement that I used was black seed oil. Black seed oil is supposed to be the God of all supplements. It's supposed to promote health across the board. They say that it's a huge anti-inflammatory and since pretty much every health problem is caused by inflammation black seed oil is probably the number one vitamin you can use. They say black seed oil is wonderful for cancer prevention and treatment. They also say it's crucial to liver health. They say that it prevents diabetes. They also say it's great for weight loss which was one of the main reasons why I started using it. They say that it's great for your hair, nails, and skin. They also say that it's wonderful for fighting off infections and that it's effective against certain strains of superbugs that most antibiotics are not working on anymore. Black seed oil has been studied over and over again. It's probably one of the most studied supplements on the market so there's some solid science to back up what it does. Still I have no idea if it had a major effect on my workout or not nor do I have any idea if it helped my weight loss.

Another supplement I used was grapeseed, green tea, and pine bark complex. The combination of these created a super antioxidant but the main reason why I was taking it was for energy. The combination of these three things promotes a natural boost in energy. It's not like a caffeine pill or anything like that it's something that works overtime. This is one of those supplements that I don't like running out of I try to make sure that I keep it in stock as much as I possibly can.

I used probiotics because they support your immune system. They're supposed to introduce positive bacteria back into your stomach, which also is supposed to help your digestive system and promote weight loss. I can say that I got sick a lot less often once I start taking the probiotics still I started sprinting around the same time so I can't really say which one was super effective against common ailments.

L-Carnitine was one of the first supplements that I started using. It aids in transforming fat into energy, which is the most important process in weight loss and energy production so I knew that I had to get L-Carnitine immediately. Also it's supposed to aid in muscle building as well. It's actually suppose to be one of the main elements of muscle building. A lot of bodybuilders use L-Carnitine and some even say it helps with your overall brain health. Now I don't know if it did any of these things for me I just know during the Sprint Diet I took it everyday.

Omega-3 fish oil is something that I've been taking since I was a kid. It's supposed to support cardiovascular health and cognitive function. Not to mention your immune system, your bone health, and your joint health as well. It's also said to support a healthy mood. I don't know if it does any of these things I just know that my mom has been giving me omega-3 fish oil since I was a kid. It's supposed to be one of the most important vitamins on the planet for preserving your body and promoting overall health.

Vitamin D3 is a supplement I started taking when I realize that I probably wasn't getting enough of it. Vitamin D comes from sun exposure and since I don't really go outside too often I knew that I probably was vitamin D3 deficient. Vitamin D3 is supposed to support bone destiny, the immune system, and boost absorption of calcium. It's supposed to support neuromuscular function whatever that means. All I know is vitamin D is very important to the body and if you're not getting enough sunlight than most likely you're not getting enough vitamin D3. Still I have no idea if it had any effect on my performance whatsoever.

Biotin is something that I also supplemented with. It's supposed to be good for your hair, nails, and skin. It's also supposed to support some other viable functions in the body. I guess biotin is one of the key ingredients that your hair needs to grow so that's one of the main reasons why I was supplementing with it. I will say when I started to use it I did notice a difference in my hair quality, nail quality, and the appearance of my skin after about maybe three to four months. Still I'm not sure if that was the sprinting or the biotin or a combination of both.

Sea kelp was something else that I used. It's supposed to be a source of iodine. Iodine is important for thyroid function. The thyroid regulates a huge amount of functions in your body including your hormonal balance. Your hormonal balance has a huge effect on your energy levels, your mood, and also your weight. If your thyroid isn't functioning properly than most likely you're going to have weight issues. They say this is why the Japanese are so skinny because their diet is rich in iodine because they eat so much seaweed. Still I have no idea if it had any effect on my weight loss.

Garcinia Cambogia is supposed to stop your body from creating new fat. It was featured on Dr. Oz a while ago and it's supposed to be proven to actually stop your body from creating new fat. Now I'm not sure if it stopped my body from creating new fat all I know is that it was a part of my everyday regimen.

Of course I took a multi vitamin because that just makes common sense. Everybody probably takes a multi-vitamin I've been taking one since I was a kid so that's always pretty much been apart of my regimen.

African Mango was also something that I included in my supplement regimen. It's supposed to help promote weight loss but there isn't much research behind it to say that it does anything of any kind of significance. Still a lot of people swear by it so I added it to my supplement pile.

 I also took L-Theanine and if you're a coffee drinker like me L-Theanine is absolutely essential. It gets rid of that jittery affect that coffee gives you and makes it a smooth high. It also has some other benefits that might be worth mentioning. Apparently in 1964 Japan approved L-Theanine for unlimited use in all foods. L-Theanine has been linked to relieving stress. It's the key ingredient in green tea, which has been linked to relieving stress.

 I'm not endorsing any of these vitamins in anyway. I'm just informing you of the supplements I used during the Sprint Diet. These supplements may have enhanced my results and it wouldn't be fair if I didn't mention them. If you choose to take them my best advice is to have a conversation with your doctor. If you want to know the exact supplements that I used than check out my website http://workoutkingrule.blogspot.com/.

Mind Your Diet

If you don't pay attention to what the f*** you eat you're not going to be able to accomplish anything. In this situation I'm speaking about eating for energy not eating for weight loss. Remember sprinting takes up a large amount of energy within the body so if you're not eating for a machine than you're not going to be able to sprint for very long. Your body is going to need power so therefore you have to eat the foods that give you the most power. I'm going to give you a detailed example of the type of foods I ate during the Sprint Diet. You can either mimic this or find similar foods that might give you the drive you need.

First thing in the morning I made sure to blend a shake. I blended kale, oranges, apples, bananas, blueberries, cranberries, strawberries, and I used apple juice instead of water. I did research on each one of these fruits and vegetables to make sure that they would give me the optimum performance that I was seeking.

Kale is the healthiest vegetable you can eat because of that I made sure to put more kale in my shake than anything else. Every single fruit that I mention I used a whole one like I used a whole orange, a whole apple, and ah whole banana. I used about maybe eight cranberries, eight blueberries, and about four strawberries. To be honest after I took the shake in the morning I always would feel wonderful. It was probably the best part of my diet and a great way to kick off my day. I also had oatmeal because I wanted to make sure that I was getting an extreme amount of fiber.

The combination of these fruits and vegetables gave me an extreme amount of energy. It's probably the one thing that I can attest to my newfound power. It actually boosts my energy level. I don't know if any of my vitamins did anything to actually boost my energy level but I'm sure my shake did the job especially in combination with oatmeal. To be honest over time it became even more effective. Most people don't understand that eating healthy is something that takes time to affect your body. Sometimes you'll be able to feel it right away but a lot of people quit because they don't feel any difference within a few days or a week. I noticed after a month of taking the shake my overall mood in general changed. Remember I told you I was a very tired, cranky, and moody individual. I was so overweight my body had absolutely no energy whatsoever. When your body has no energy it pretty much ruins everything. You don't want to do anything. I can say that this shake had a profound effect on that mindset and was a key ingredient in making the Sprint Diet much more effective. I made sure that I didn't add any sugar to the mix and I also made sure to put cinnamon in my oatmeal and I found out that actually had a profound effect or my health as well. Remember cinnamon is nothing but pure fiber and fiber is incredibly important to the digestive system. As long as you're going to the bathroom often you're losing weight so you want to make sure you're getting as much fiber as you possibly can. That's why I added apples to the mix because apples are rich in fiber. It's also why I added blueberries to the mix because they're rich in fiber as well. I wanted to make sure that I upped my fiber intake by as much as I possibly could. I also wanted to make sure I was getting a ton of vitamin C.

Vitamin C is the reason why I made sure to add a whole Orange. I added bananas to the mix because I wanted to make sure that I was getting a lot of potassium but really I wanted the bananas for the Vitamin B6. Vitamin B6 is something that you'll see in almost every natural energy supplement.

Cranberries were just another source of fiber they have even more fiber than blueberries they're also packed full of antioxidants. The strawberries were mostly for flavor at first until I started doing more research and I realize that strawberries were amazing. They can help prevent heart disease, stroke, cancer, high blood pressure, constipation, allergies, asthma diabetes, and depression. Strawberries are ah incredibly effective antioxidant.

Oatmeal is packed full of iron it's probably one of the most iron rich foods out there. It also has an extremely large amount of vitamin B6, magnesium, and vitamin A not to mention 6 grams of protein. Speaking of protein maybe I should discuss what I had for lunch.

Everyday for lunch I would have grilled chicken, beans, and a protein shake. My lunch was all about protein intake. At lunch time I wanted to make sure that I was getting as much protein in my body as possible that's why I made sure I had grilled chicken because chicken has an extremely large amount of protein. Chicken is one of the most protein rich meats on the planet and it's healthier for you than beef or pork. Not to mention it's a lot easier to cook especially if you know how to bake or if you have a griller like one of those commercial grillers that drain out all the grease. Everyday when I woke up in the morning I would make sure that I put on my rice cooker and I would add one cup or two cups of black beans. I chose black beans because they're low in calories. One cup is only 624 calories and because they are extremely high in dietary fiber, you get 29 grams in one cup. Also because they're high in protein you get 39 grams of protein in one cup. They have an extremely large amount of iron, and ah extremely large amount of magnesium, and calcium so it was an obvious choice. Black beans are a incredibly healthy super food with 2760 mg of potassium.

The body is supposed to consume at least 30 to 38 grams of fiber every day if you're a man. If you're a woman it's about 25 grams of fiber everyday. So basically one cup of black beans would almost be enough fiber for the day for a man and more than enough for a woman. If you read up on black beans you'll understand just how nutritious they really are. It's one of the most underestimated super foods on the planet. The only substitute that I would ever use for black beans if I didn't have them is quinoa because it's probably the greatest food on the planet and the only food that has pretty much all the amino acids that you need.

I made sure that I had a whey protein isolate shake everyday. Since sprinting increases protein synthesis by 230 percent. Consuming ah s*** ton of protein and sprinting is genius. It's a final trump card to make sure that your body is burning fat and building muscle

For dinner I ate pretty much anything I wanted I just made sure that I didn't eat any fast food. I completely cut out fast food in general. For dinner I would have a meal with black beans on the side. I would have ground turkey meat, chicken, or fish. I wouldn't have any beef or pork. So I would have some turkey tacos with black beans, and cheese, or I would have some turkey nachos with black beans, and cheese. Sometimes I would eat some salmon, beans, and rice. As long as I added the black beans to the meal I would pretty much create any combination I wanted. Eating beans with your meal helps the digestive process not to mention it increases the nutritional value of the meal. I didn't really eat any dessert but I've never been one to eat dessert anyway so it wasn't a big change for me.

My diet wasn't too extreme it wasn't anything that was impractical. All my food was good it wasn't like I had to eat nasty s*** that I didn't like. When you have to eat a bunch of nasty s*** that you don't like eventually you're going to give up on it. I loved the s*** I was eating! My shake was delicious and my oatmeal was always good especially once I added cinnamon. I never put sugar in my oatmeal I just added cinnamon to it. If I wanted it to taste good I would add some honey. I made sure that I got my honey from the whole food store so that my s*** was natural. I didn't mind the beans I was eating because I was eating black beans and those are my favorite especially once you season them with some Lawry's and some pepper. The grilled chicken was always good because I mean grilled chicken is f****** awesome. Sometimes I would grill chicken and have a chicken black bean salad. That s*** was good. My diet gave me energy, power, and change my mood all together. It's the main reason why I was able to go on. If I never changed my diet I would have never saw any positive effects from the Sprint Diet in the first place because I wouldn't be able to do it. My intention was never to change my diet for weight loss but to promote energy production. I simply wanted to feel better and run longer and this diet accomplished that for me. I didn't find it difficult. If you can find food that has similar nutritious value that you actually find delicious by all means go about it in your own way. I'm just telling you exactly what I did I don't want to leave any details out because that might be the one detail that contributed to my progression. If you choose to follow my diet to the letter it is more likely that you will see the same results that I did. Maybe you might find some loopholes that I didn't find and you might be able to improve upon the diet. If so please don't hoard information comment and add your perspective. Tell the people of the dietary changes you implement that worked in combination with the Sprint Diet or maybe some of the vitamins that you used in combination with the Sprint Diet. Share other forms of sprinting that you tried in combination with the Sprint Diet that worked for you.

In Conclusion

Throughout my workout journey I tried everything in extremes. Some days I would get on the bike for an hour. Than after that I would get on the treadmill for an hour. Than after that I would get on the elliptical for an hour. I did this for months with no results. I decided to get on the elliptical for 3 hours a day making sure that I burned 3000 calories every single day. I did that for a month with no major results. I decided to up the ante and add an extra hour to the equation making sure that I was burning 3500 calories a day and after a month of doing that I saw absolutely no results. 3500 calories is a pound and I wasn't over eating in any way whatsoever. I even boosted it up to five hours on the elliptical everyday and still I got no results. I got so used to doing extended aerobic exercise that I had the energy of a marathon runner. As far as my stamina was concerned my normal day-to-day energy was still low but my ability to keep going on the elliptical machine was impressive yet it got me no major results. I was doing five hours on the elliptical machine burning upwards of 4200 calories and still I saw no results. If I was doing that much work and still not seeing any results imagine ah individual who comes in the gym and does 30 minutes on the bike every single day expecting to see major results. Imagine ah individual who comes in and walks on the treadmill for 45 minutes to an hour and expects to see major results. Imagine someone who comes in and uses the elliptical for an hour and expects to see major results it's unfathomable it's a fantasy. None of those people truly are going to lose any weight. I was out doing everyone in my gym. People were asking me how long I was on the machine because others would tell them that I was there when they arrived and I was there when they left. I was there all day and all night because I was serious about my weight loss. Still it had absolutely no major effects whatsoever the only thing it did was give me the ability to run from one city to the next without getting tired but my body still looked horrible. What's the point of gaining long-term stamina if your body still looks like s***? It was a complete and utter waste of time. If I would have just sprinted from the very beginning I would've had even more stamina long-term, short-term, and day-to-day energy. Not to mention muscle and actually physically visible results, which is what I really, wanted. I wanted physically visible results and that's what sprinting gave me. I could look in the mirror and actually see the inches drop off of me. When I was on the elliptical machine and all the other machines for hours upon hours the only thing I would do is weigh myself on the scale once every 7 days. Admittedly this is a mistake never count on a scale to measure how much you weigh because a scale does not account for how much of your body is muscle and how much of your body is fat and how much of your body is water so it's going to be off it's always going to be off. You measure your weight loss in inches. Get a measuring tape and measure your waistline. The smaller your waist gets the more weight you actually lost and the more muscle you've added to your body. This is a lesson I also had to learn the hard way. Aerobic exercise is good for long-term stamina but it's not efficient at burning fat trust me on this. Like I said before have you ever noticed any of those people that only use the aerobic machines actually lose major weight? Those machines are ancient they've been around since the inception of the gym yet no one speaks of there results being godlike. If those machines were super effective the gym would be much more popular than it is. The most powerful workout tool is sprinting. If more people were sprinting everyday than we would have a much healthier society. Everyone would have much more energy and everyone would waste a lot less time at the gym. I wasted months at the gym trying to push my body as far as I possibly could. I would test the limits of my abilities every single day and yes I was capable of running longer every day but when I looked in the mirror I was looking at the same man. It was frustrating as fuck! To be honest if I wasn't as stubborn as I was I would have stopped doing it a long time ago. The day I discovered sprinting was the day everything changed. From the first run I already knew that this was a type of exercise that really would have a true impact on my weight loss. I knew this type of exercise was going to change the way I felt every day. It's the one type of exercise that I actually respect because I know it's working. I can feel that it is working. I can feel the fatigue. I can feel the endorphins running around in my head. I can feel the rush of dopamine. I can feel my body trying to replenish itself after being taxed to its maximum limit. After every week I could feel the difference in my energy level. This made me feel like I was actually doing something for the first time. I know that sounds crazy because I used to run on an elliptical machine for 5 hours straight but it never taxed my body the way sprinting for 2 minutes did. It was amazing to think that I could move on an elliptical machine with the difficulty turned up almost to max for 5 hours but I could barely sprint 6 times for 10 seconds. This one form of exercise completely changed my life. Everything that I considered motivation for doing this exercise was eventually accomplished. I've never felt better about myself as a person and I've never felt more like I'm the s*** than I do now. Every single day when I get up and look in the mirror I feel like I'm the s***! That doesn't mean that I knock others down or belittle them because I know how it feels to be unconfident and doubtful of your own self-worth. That's why I wrote this book to help people that are doubtful and uncertain of their own self-worth. I wrote this book for people that are on the borderline of giving up because they have tried for so long and have seen absolutely no results whatsoever. It could seem at some point that it's not meant for you to lose weight like your body will never change. That's how I felt before I begun the Sprint Diet. My pre-diabetic status, my high blood pressure, and my low energy all eventually went away by following the principles in this book. If this information can help even one person than it was worth writing down. I've seen tons of information on dieting and exercise throughout the Internet but none of those things helped me. Some people have been skinny their entire lives and than out of nowhere gained a ton of weight and they don't know how to manage it. Weight management is just something that they never had to deal with because their weight was never a concern. Some people have been big their whole life but have never really tried to do anything about it so when they do try they go through this whole list of things that make absolutely no difference. Throughout my journey I listen to many people I took many routes and every one of them led me down the same path. The worst feeling in the world is working as hard as you possibly can at something but literally getting nowhere. It's like the universe is saying your best isn't enough. In the case of exercise it's not that your best isn't enough it's just that you're giving your all to the wrong things. I gave my all to every single form of aerobic exercise you can imagine. Hours every day non-stop spent working out with minimal to no results. Once I gave my all to sprinting I finally could see the fruits of my labor. I finally felt like I actually was doing something productive something beneficial that was pushing past the threshold that I had been at for months. Remember nothing is instantaneous everything takes time but the worst thing you can do is waste your time doing something that isn't beneficial. I'm glad I went down the path I did because now I can invite others to take an alternative route. When I go into the gym and I see people that I know using the treadmill or the elliptical I make sure to inform them that there is an alternative method something more beneficial. I tell them about sprinting and they always think me later. Still I never really felt like I was reaching enough people that way and hopefully through this book I can reach out to people that felt just like I did, willing to make a change but oblivious of how to go about it. We all want to make a change but most of us don't know how to go about it so when we try for the first time and fail some of us never try again. If this is your first time trying to lose weight and become healthy than I'm glad you came here first. Have a good workout and ah energetic and long life.

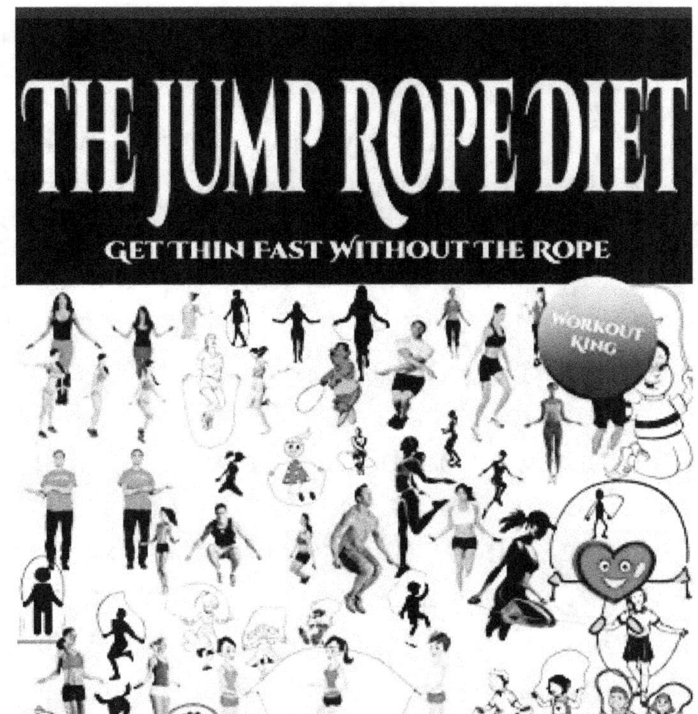

The Jump Rope Diet

This Is My Story

My story isn't anything special. My doctor told me I would be a pre-diabetic if I didn't lose weight. Naturally I was a little ashamed because I was a young man at the time. Surprisingly no one told me I had a weight problem. For some reason I was oblivious to it. Looking back on my pictures now I think to myself how didn't I see it. Sometimes we get so comfortable with our bad habits that we don't even see the negative effects. It's similar to how an alcoholic can't see how he's harming himself, and everyone around him. It's similar to how a drug addict can't see that his addiction is deteriorating his appearance.

The day my doctor told me I was in danger of becoming a diabetic changed my life. On that day I decided that my health was more important than my cravings. I decided that my health was more important than my comfortable laziness. Comfort is a funny thing because comfort creates habits. I was comfortable with my negative habits because of that I sacrificed my health. Finding out I was going to be a diabetic was very painful for me. I remember as a child watching my grandmother die of diabetes. I promised her I would take care of myself. I felt like I let her down. I had to do something about my health. I had to do something about my mindset.

In the course of watching some positive, and uplifting videos I came across Muhammad Ali training. I saw his intensity with the jump rope, and I admired it. I could see his speed, and coordination came from his jump roping. Jump roping gave him his ability to dodge so easily. It was the reason he could float like a butterfly, and sting like ah bee. I decided to give it a try. Really what did I have to lose? I immediately figured out that I was no good at it. I loved the workout, but I hated the Rope. I felt like the rope was unnecessary. The majority of the workout is calves, and ankles. So I decided to do a little research to see if it would matter or not if I remove the rope from the equation. Turns out it's not a very big deal as long as you have something in your hand that's just as heavy as the rope handle. I used hand grippers. You've probably seen them before. Just in case you haven't here's a picture.

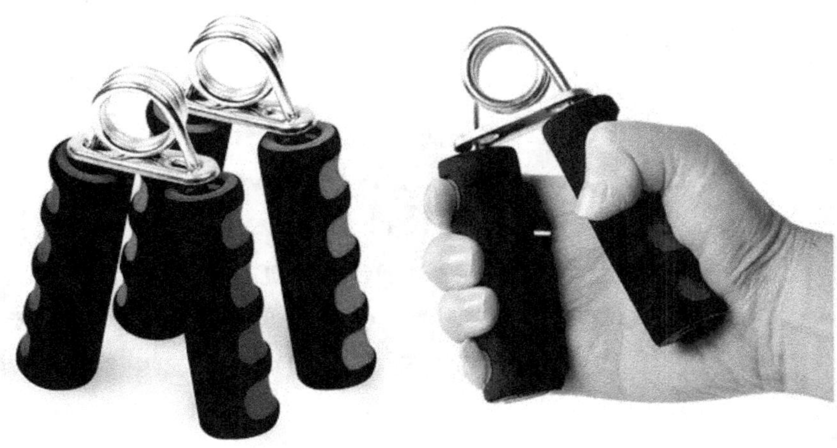

I grab one of the handles on each hand gripper an act like I'm spinning a rope. I even time my jump as if a rope is actually coming down. This exercise helped me burn so much fat in such a short period of time. It's such an easy exercise to do. It's very difficult for me to make excuses not to do it. Plus I couldn't argue with the results. Without the jump rope diet I would have never lost the weight. To believe that something I used to do in Elementary would benefit me later on in life. It was quite surprising to me that I never thought to do it before. I mean if I jumped from the beginning I would've never gained weight in the first place.

I jumped rope for about three to four months. I went to see my doctor, and I got a clean bill of health. I felt like I accomplished something. Even getting my high school diploma, and college degree didn't affect me like that did. This accomplishment felt spiritual mental, and physical. It was such a crazy combination of emotions to hear that news. My wife was proud of me, and I was proud of her. We did this together. When we started we were just dating, and after it was done we were married. I think the journey connected us, and that's why I recommend that you do this with someone else. It doesn't have to be a girlfriend or boyfriend, but the camaraderie really increases everyone's focus.

That was some time ago jump roping has been a part of my life for years now. It's something I do everyday. I should say it's something my wife, and I do everyday. <u>The Jump Rope Diet</u> has been amazing for us, and I know it's going to be amazing for you.

The Benefits Of Jumping Rope

Jump roping Burns anywhere from 10 to 16 calories per minute. Yes I said 10 to 16 calories per minute! That's absolutely astounding! If you keep a steady pace, and really push yourself you can burn a thousand calories every hour using the jump rope. With <u>The Jump Rope Diet</u> you don't have to use an actual jump rope. It's a lot easier to continue to work out when you don't have to worry about the rope smacking up against your legs. You're more worried about actually jumping so you can focus.

10 minutes of jump roping is equivalent to ah 8-minute mile. That's absolutely crazy when you

think about it. We're talking about a playground exercised out doing the mile run one of the most famous forms of training there is. The mile run is going to put extreme stress on your joints, and it's going to be insanely tiring. Jump roping for 10 minutes isn't going to be nearly as brutal, but just as effective. The American Heart Association has placed its whole movement around jumping rope. Everyone's heard of Jump Rope for Heart. When it comes to the fight against heart disease no exercise is more effective than jumping rope. Jump roping gets your heart rate up everyone knows this. Jump roping promotes a healthy blood flow, and lowers your cholesterol. Jump roping prevents heart disease, and stroke two illnesses that take out some of our best, and brightest. Jump roping strengthens the connection between your body, and your brain. You're jumping on the balls of your feet so your mind has to make neuromuscular adjustments. It does this to make sure that you remain balanced. As this connection gets stronger your body reacts quicker to different situations. It increases the speed in which signals between the body, and the mind can be sent causing you to have quicker reflexes. This is why boxers jump rope because they want to increase their reflexes. Boxes need to be able to move out of the way at any given point in time to avoid injury. By jump roping they develop a strong connection between body and mind. This is why the best boxers in the world are some of the most hardcore jump ropers. Muhammad Ali, and Floyd Mayweather are two of the greatest defensive fighters ever, and they're amazing jump ropers.

Jump roping is great for increasing bone density. Most people think jump roping has a hard impact on your joints, and bones. Jump roping is far less impactful than running. That's because you're landing on both feet. When you run you land on one foot. This puts all the force on one leg. When you jump rope both legs are absorbing the force. Also you're not coming nearly as high off the ground. I only jump an inch to in half an inch off the ground. It's really about the surface that you're jumping on more than anything. I don't jump on concrete. I don't jump on grass. I don't jump on wood! I only jump on carpet with my folded yoga mat under me. I make the surface as soft as I possibly can. I've never had a problem with my knees, ankles, or hips.

Before you start <u>The Jump Rope Diet</u> make sure you do some reverse calf raises. Build strength in the muscles most impacted by jump roping. Most likely those muscles are going to be very weak which is where the initial soreness is going to come from. That's why it's good to isolate, and work those muscles with calf raises, and reverse calf raises.

The Jump Rope Diet zaps weight off your body while increasing your focus, and coordination. When you take the rope out of the situation it's an extremely easy exercise. It's something you can do anywhere with virtually zero equipment. Without the rope you don't have to worry about hitting things or knocking things over. You only need body space. You can do it anywhere that has enough space for you to jump an inch to a half an inch off the ground. This made it very easy for me, and my wife. We were able to travel, and go wherever we wanted to without worrying about having enough space to exercise. We literally could exercise in the shower if we wanted to. Not that we did, but we could have. The shower has plenty space for The Jump Rope Diet.

Beginners

I'm going to tell you everything that I did in detail. I'll try to make sure I don't leave anything out. Even the smallest details are going to be mentioned so just bear with me. Every morning my wife would get up, and put on motivational workout videos. For some reason those videos motivate her. I'm not talking about videos where people are taking you through a designated workout. It was just a mixture of female fitness models training. At first I didn't really get it, but eventually it did end up motivating me. Something about watching those girls really commit to extreme fitness like CrossFit was motivational. So I didn't bother my wife about it. Now days even when she's not with me I still watch the videos.

Next I fill up a gallon of water. That's right I said a gallon of water! This kind of exercise is going to require you to stay extremely hydrated.

Next I grab my yoga mat, and lay down on the carpet folding it in half.

Next I grabbed my hand grippers.

Now I do this with my socks on I don't wear shoes, but you can if you want. When I was on a beginner level I set my timer to 15 minutes I pressed go, and started jumping as fast as I could. I made sure I only came an inch to ah half an inch off the mat. I have perfect posture making sure not to lean forward or backward. I kept my hands at my side, and I move the hand grippers like I was holding a jump rope. Sometimes I would grab both handles on the hand grippers, and start squeezing them to get a quick wrist, and forearm workout while keeping the turning motion. I would squeeze it about 50 times.

When the timer hit 30 seconds I would stop. Eventually I was able to work myself up to one minute which is what I consider beginner level. When you begin training do 30 sets of 30-second jumps that's 15 minutes. When you gain more stamina you'll go up to 30 sets of one-minute jumps for 30 minutes of exercise. That's what I consider beginner level training. If you can jump longer than by all means do so. Most people will start off on this level. They won't be able to do one-minute jumps right away. If you're the exception than be proud of yourself for an excellent start. Throughout the entire exercise you want to squeeze your core. You'll increase your balance, strengthen your core, and drop some unwanted belly fat. Once again I'll reiterate make sure that you drink water.

Another thing to consider is to stretch out your calves, and ankles. I'll leave some photos of some stretches you can do below.

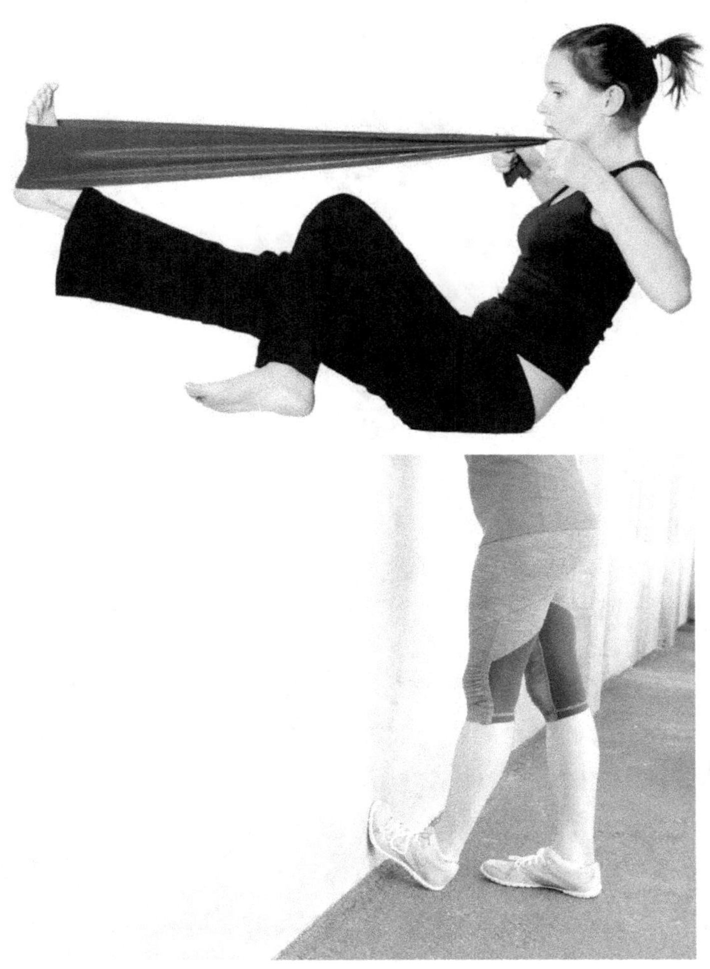

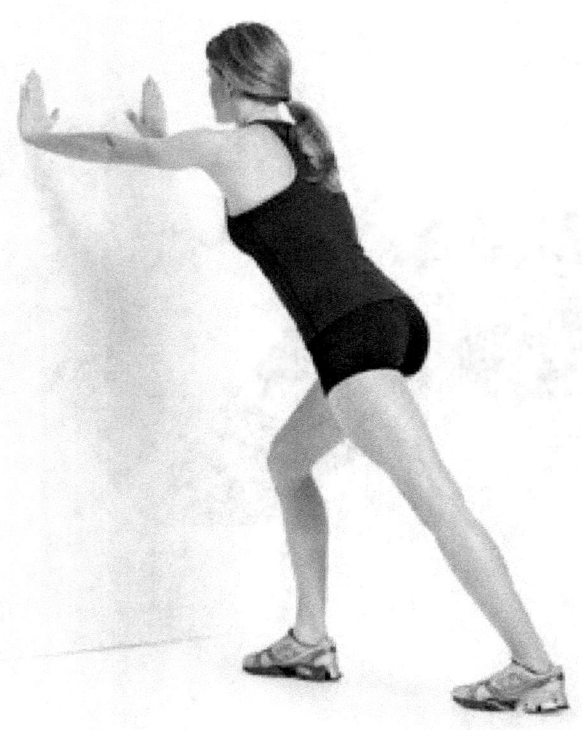

These muscles are slightly temperamental
because they're not often worked. That's why you
need to stretch, and work them. Your ankles hold
up your entire body so you want them to be as
strong as iron. For the life of me I can't think of an
exercise that works the ankles better than jump
roping.

Intermediate

The intermediate program has two steps. Step one start doing an hour of jump roping. Step 2; get your jump time up to two minutes per set. The first thing I did was up my time to 45 minutes. I also upped my jump time to a minute, and 30 seconds. I did this for about 10 to 15 days. Eventually my body adjusted to it, and it was easy for me. I up my time to an hour while still doing one minute, and 30 seconds each set. After about 5 days of this I was able to do 2 minutes each set.

This is the way I went about doing it you can pretty much go about upping your time anyway you want. Grow at your own pace. These are just guidelines you don't have to follow them exactly. The point is to improve. I just want to be very specific about how I went about improving. I found it was easier to increase the time of the session then it was to increase the time of the set. I also found out increasing the time of the session builds up stamina increasing the time of my set. Instead of doing 30 minutes of jump roping one minute each set I could go up to 45 minutes 1 minute each set. Eventually that would get me strong enough to do 1:30 seconds each set.

When I started doing 30 sets of 2-minute jumps everything changed. I started to notice my results come in a lot faster. I started to notice my face slim down, and my waist start to drop. I felt more focused I felt more involved in the exercise. Usually when I exercise I feel like I'm not in the moment. I don't really know how to explain it but I'm pretty sure everyone else will agree with me. Once I got to this point in the jump rope diet I felt in the moment. I was focused, and prepared for the workout. Once I felt that feeling I started to understand why boxers seemed to enjoy this work out so much. It's truly a shared experience between the body, and the mind. That's just my personal opinion I'll let you be the judge.

My wife was especially focused. Usually she's the last one up in the morning but when we reach this point in our training she just had this energy about her. Up and ready before I could even turn the alarm off. That's when I knew we were onto something. After two months the physical results weren't staggering, but we felt sensational. I've never seen my wife have so much energy. Once you reach this point you're ready for advanced level training.

Advance

Things are about to get interesting. When you hit an advanced level it means that you're capable of doing an hour of jump roping three minutes per set. You'll be doing twenty sets 3 minutes each. Now some people go higher honestly I've never done more than a five-minute set. I wouldn't recommend anything more. Even though a man once jumped rope for 36 hours straight with no major issues I'd still be cautious. No one on the planet is as good as Mark Rothstein when it comes to jumping rope.

Now your body is strong, and it requires more resistance. This is where leg weights come in. Now I always say be very careful with leg weights when you're doing cardio exercises. You don't want leg weights that are incredibly loose because it will cause problems. My recommendation would be no more than 5 pounds on each leg. If you can find some leg weights that are well insulated, and don't move around when you jump you can put more weight on. Unfortunately I personally haven't come across any leg weights that fit that description. Leg weights will send you all the way back to the beginning. Most likely you'll have to do 30 seconds to one-minute sets. Continue to do, and our overall, but be aware that you're set time we'll go down at first. If you can't do an hour do 30 minutes. My set time went down to about a minute when I put 5 pounds on each leg. It was the same with my wife she put 2.5 pounds on each leg. That's what I would recommend for women depending on how strong your legs are. The leg weights make you feel like a beginner all over again, and I love that feeling. It means that the results are going to be amazing, and they were. Adding the leg weights to the workout severely improved my results. Little by little I was able to work back up to 3-minute sets with 10 pounds on my legs.

At this point my wife made a really smart purchase, and bought us some wrist weights. She got 2.5 pounds for each hand. Now we were jumping with 15 extra pounds on us. This brought me down to 2 minutes per set. It didn't take me long to build back up to 3 minutes sets.

If that isn't enough for you than I have a killer of an idea. Why don't you put on a weight vest? This is exactly what my wife said to me right before we bought a 20-pound weight vest. That weight vest changed my life. Once I started jumping with the weight vests on those pounds just dropped off. At first I would only wear the weight vests, and the wrist weights for a total of 25 pounds. This of course took me back to one-minute jumps all over again. With resilience I was able to work back up to 3-minute jumps, and I never felt better.

I remember looking in the mirror, and seeing a totally different guy. It was like I finally broke the mold. I felt like I was stuck for so long so when

I got to this point I couldn't do anything, but be proud of myself. No matter how hard the universe tried a negative thought couldn't ruin the moment. I had taken back control. After that feeling I just wanted to up the weight one last time, and add ankle weights in for a total of 35 pounds. Once again I had to go back to one-minute jumps, but I work my way up again.

Another way to increase the resistance is to jump on sand. Not only does it reduce the impact significantly it also makes it more difficult for you to jump. The added resistance makes for a much better workout, and a much safer one. If you add all the extra weight, and jump in the sand you're on a whole new level. Be careful with the weight make sure you don't add more than you can handle. This exercise increases your results significantly, but it's also risky if you're not strong enough. Give your body rest, and make sure you stretch, and keep good form.

Adding the weight helps you build muscle, and burn way more calories. It really made the difference in my training. It's the reason why I was able to lose so much weight. It took a simple exercise, and turned it into weighted cardio.

Motivation

No plan succeeds without motivation. Motivation is the foundation of every major come up or comeback. For some people motivation is like an hourglass eventually all the sand will fall to the bottom. At that point all your motivation will be gone. If that's the case you need to make sure that there's enough sand in that hourglass to carry you to the end.

You need to start off with extreme a amount of motivation. Overtime different things will end up motivating you to push forward. Not only physical results, but also mental results as well. The way that you feel will change which will also motivate you. It might be some time before these results show themselves so you need to have at least 3 months of motivation built up in you before you start this journey. 3 months is long enough to see some results that will than motivate you further. Some people start off a weight loss regimen with only a week's worth of motivation. That's not nearly enough to see any major results. I've heard individuals tell me that I worked out for 2 weeks straight, and didn't see any results. Of course you didn't see any results two weeks isn't nearly enough time for a person to see physical change. That's why I encourage you now to build up as much motivation as you possibly can. You need to understand that some days you're going to wake up, and not want to do this. Some days you're going to wake up, and feel drained, and tired.

Different life circumstances, and events could happen in the middle of your journey. Ah death could occur in your family. A difficult task could come up. A difficult work situation could strain you. You might even lose your job. Through all of this you need to remain motivated, and continue putting your health first. All those things are important, but what's most important is you. For once put yourself first. The best way to put yourself first is to put your health first. Putting your health first is putting your life on a pedestal just a little quote from my wife.

A lot could happen in a three-month time span so beware of the distractions. People mention the small distractions, but it's really the big ones that give people the excuse to stop. If something dramatic happens in their life they feel like it's a big enough excuse for them to stop putting themselves first. For me it was a matter of learning how to cope with different problems in my life through Fitness. Every time something negative would happen in my life I would deal with it by working out. I was able to think clearly on the situation, and make better decisions that way. When you work out your brain works better so you're better capable of dealing with your emotions.

I remember right in the mist of the jump rope diet my grandma died. Now usually an event like this would cause me to backtrack. I remembered what my grandma on my mom's side said to me. She wanted me to take care of myself so that I could live a better life than she did. I know that's exactly what my grandma on my dad's side would have wanted as well. If she knew that I had stopped my fitness she would be upset with me so I continued. More challenging events occurred during this time like me losing my job. Still even during my unemployment I continued my fitness.

My fitness is actually the reason I was able to work a new job. My wife, and I were at the gym jump roping on some yoga mats without the rope when a gentleman approaches us. He wanted to know what we were doing he had never seen anyone jump rope without the rope. Eventually he joined us, and we became great friends. It was through him that I was able to get a new job, and a new workout buddy. Working out is good for keeping a positive mindset that's why it's good to continue your fitness when you're in a negative situation. So no matter what's going on in your life get up grab a friend, and jump.

My motivation was especially high. At no point did I believe giving up was an option. Giving up to me was giving up on my life. My physician made it very clear that if I didn't start taking care of myself I was going to become a diabetic. There was no way I wanted to live like that. The choice was continue being lazy, and become a diabetic, and potentially die or take care of myself, and live a long healthy life. It was pretty much a no-brainer for me. I hope the decision is as clear cut, and dry for you as it was for me. If not you need to find other reasons to be motivated.

Sometimes vanity isn't enough. Most individuals want to get in shape so they can look good, but sometimes that isn't enough. I should say most of the time that isn't enough. That's usually the reason why a lot of people end up in the gym. They want to improve their physical appearance so it has nothing to do with their health. Those who usually stay in the gym are those who are concerned about their health. When you're doing it for vain reasons than your motivation quickly relies on your vanity. If you're not a very vain person then your motivation is going to run out quickly. If you are a very vain individual than your motivation might last a lot longer.

Vanity can be a part of your motivation, but it shouldn't be the driving force. Think about your health, and all the love ones you'll leave behind. Think about your children if you have them. Think about your significant other, and how they'll feel when your health starts to take a turn for the worse. These are solid reasons to be motivated. In my opinion the greatest source of motivation is someone who is just as determined as you are. Having friends to do this with is a powerful source of motivation. If you can get everyone together, and create a sense of camaraderie there's nothing you can't accomplish.

The sense of camaraderie that my wife, and I had is one of the main reasons we were able to finish, and continue our training. If I didn't want to do it she would make me do it. If she didn't want to do it I would make her do it. Eventually we didn't even have to motivate each other anymore it was just second nature. We were going to get up, and we were going to work out. Once it gets to that point you can't lose because now it's a part of your permanent routine like coffee in the morning.

All you need to do is find out how many calories your body needs to maintain its current weight. Eat 500 less calories than that every day. Couple that with the jump rope diet, and you'll be fine.

Vitamin Intake

Let me start this off by saying that by no means am I telling you to buy any of these vitamins. I'm just telling you the vitamins that I used during The Jump Rope Diet. I have no idea if they had an effect on my results, but I feel like they're worth mentioning. My vitamin intake during The Jump Rope Diet was well rounded. I tried to make sure I covered every single function of my body. Let's start things off with the first vitamin I took.

Ubiquinol is said to be very good for your cardiovascular health, and the last thing I wanted going out on me was my heart because I had high blood pressure. Ubiquinol was a supplement I took to make sure I had a little extra energy. Its supposed to be an incredibly powerful antioxidant it's also supposed to promote energy production as well, and I needed all the energy that I could get. They say it's good for brain health, and protecting the cells from free radicals. To be honest I still use ubiquinol it's much better than Co q-10 because it's easily absorb into the body.

The second thing I kind of supplemented with was <u>Apple Cider Vinegar With Mother</u>. I mixed my apple cider vinegar with a teaspoon of lemon juice, eight ounces of water, and made sure to take this every single day at least 2 times a day. I have no idea what kind of effect it may have had on my progression. I just know that it's still apart of my routine to this day. Apple cider vinegar is supposed to promote weight loss. I have no idea if it contributed to my weight loss, but I feel like it's worth mentioning.

The third supplement that I used was <u>Black Seed Oil</u>. Black seed oil is supposed to be the God of all supplements. It's supposed to promote health across the board. They say that it's a huge anti-inflammatory. Since pretty much every health problem is caused by inflammation black seed oil is probably the number one vitamin you can use. They say black seed oil is wonderful for cancer prevention, and treatment. They also say it's crucial to liver health. They say that it prevents diabetes. They also say it's great for weight loss which was one of the main reasons why I started using it. They say that it's great for your hair, nails, and skin. They also say that it's wonderful for fighting off infections, and that it's effective against certain strains of superbugs that most antibiotics are not working on anymore. Black seed oil has been studied over, and over again. It's probably one of the most studied supplements on the market so there's some solid science to back up what it does. Still I have no idea if it had a major effect on my workout or not nor do I have any idea if it helped my weight loss.

Another supplement I used was <u>Grapeseed, Green Tea, & Pine Bark Complex</u>. The combination of these creates a super antioxidant. The main reason why I was taking it was for energy. The combination of these three things promotes a natural boost in energy. It's not like a caffeine pill or anything like that it's something that works overtime. This is one of those supplements that I don't like running out of I try to make sure that I keep it in stock as much as I possibly can.

I used <u>Probiotics</u> because they support your immune system. They're supposed to introduce positive bacteria back into your stomach. This is supposed to help your digestive system, and promote weight loss. I can say that I got sick a lot less often once I start taking the probiotics. Still I started sprinting around the same time so I can't really say which one was super effective.

L-Carnitine was one of the first supplements that I started using. It aids in transforming fat into energy. This is the most important process in weight loss, and energy production. Also it's supposed to aid in muscle building as well. It's supposed to be one of the main elements of muscle building. A lot of bodybuilders use L-Carnitine, and some even say it helps with your overall brain health. Now I don't know if it did any of these things for me I just know during The Jump Rope Diet I took it everyday.

Omega-3 Fish Oil is something that I've been taking since I was a kid. It's supposed to support cardiovascular health, and cognitive function. It supports your immune system, your bone health, and your joint health as well. It's also said to support a healthy mood. I don't know if it does any of these things I just know that my mom has been giving me omega-3 fish oil since I was a kid. It's supposed to be one of the most important vitamins on the planet for preserving your body, and promoting overall health.

Vitamin D3 is a supplement I started taking when I realize that I probably wasn't getting enough of it. Vitamin D comes from sun exposure, and since I don't really go outside too often I knew that I probably was vitamin D3 deficient. Vitamin D3 is supposed to support bone destiny, the immune system, and boost absorption of calcium. It's supposed to support neuromuscular function whatever that means. All I know is Vitamin D3 is very important to the body, and if you're not getting enough sunlight than most likely you're not getting enough vitamin D3. Still I have no idea if it had any effect on my performance whatsoever.

    <u>Biotin</u> is something that I also supplemented with. It's supposed to be good for your hair, nails, and skin. It's also supposed to support some other viable functions in the body. I guess biotin is one of the key ingredients that your hair needs to grow. That's one of the main reasons why I was supplementing with it. I will say when I started to use it I did notice a difference in quality in my hair, nails, and the appearance of my skin. It took about three to four months though. Still I'm not sure if that was <u>The Jump Rope Diet</u> or the biotin or a combination of both.

    <u>Sea kelp</u> was something else that I used. It's supposed to be a source of iodine. Iodine is important for thyroid function. The thyroid

regulates a huge amount of functions in your body including your hormonal balance. Your hormonal balance has a huge effect on your energy levels, your mood, and also your weight. If your thyroid isn't functioning properly than most likely you're going to have weight issues. They say this is why the Japanese are so skinny because their diet is rich in iodine. It's because they eat so much seaweed. Still I have no idea if it had any effect on my weight loss.

Garcinia Cambogia is supposed to stop your body from creating new fat. It was featured on Dr. Oz a while ago, and it's supposed to be proven to actually stop your body from creating new fat. Now I'm not sure if it stopped my body from creating new fat all I know is that it was a part of my everyday regimen.

Of course I took a Multi Vitamin because that just makes common sense. Everybody probably takes a multi-vitamin I've been taking one since I was a kid. It's always been apart of my regimen.

African Mango was also something that I included in my supplement regimen. It's supposed to help promote weight loss but there isn't much research behind it to say that it does anything of any kind of significance. Still a lot of people swear by it so I added it to my supplement pile.

I also took <u>L-Theanine</u>, and if you're a coffee drinker like me L-Theanine is absolutely essential. It gets rid of that jittery affect that coffee gives you, and makes it a smooth high. It also has some other benefits that might be worth mentioning. Apparently in 1964 Japan approved L-Theanine for unlimited use in all foods. L-Theanine has been linked to relieving stress. It's the key ingredient in green tea, which has been linked to relieving stress.

I'm not endorsing any of these vitamins in anyway. I'm just informing you of the supplements I used during <u>The Jump Rope Diet.</u> These supplements may have enhanced my results, and it wouldn't be fair if I didn't mention them. If you choose to take them my best advice is to have a conversation with your doctor. If you want to know the exact supplements that I used than check out my website http://workoutkingrule.blogspot.com/.

Mind Your Diet

If you don't pay attention to what you eat you're not going to be able to accomplish anything. In this situation I'm speaking about eating for energy not eating for weight loss. Remember <u>The Jump Rope Diet</u> takes a lot of energy. If you're not eating for energy than you're not going to be able to last for very long. Your body is going to need power so therefore you have to eat the foods that give you the most power. I'm going to give you a detailed example of the type of foods I ate during <u>The Jump Rope Diet</u>. You can either mimic this, or find similar foods that might give you the drive you need.

First thing in the morning I made sure to blend a shake. I blended kale, oranges, apples, bananas, blueberries, cranberries, strawberries, and I used apple juice instead of water. I did research on each one of these fruits, and vegetables to make sure that they would give me the optimum performance that I was seeking.

Kale is the healthiest vegetable you can eat. I made sure to put more kale in my shake than anything else. Every single fruit that I mention I used a whole one. I used a whole orange, a whole apple, and ah whole banana. I used about maybe eight cranberries, eight blueberries, and about four strawberries. To be honest after I took the shake in the morning I always would feel wonderful. It was probably the best part of my diet, and a great way to kick off my day. I also had oatmeal because I wanted to make sure that I was getting an extreme amount of fiber.

The combination of these fruits and vegetables gave me an extreme amount of energy. It's probably the one thing that I can attest to my newfound power. It actually boosts my energy level. I don't know if any of my vitamins did anything to actually boost my energy level, but I'm sure my shake did the job. To be honest over time it became even more effective. Most people don't understand that eating healthy is something that takes time to affect your body. Sometimes you'll be able to feel it right away, but a lot of people quit because they don't feel any difference within a few days, or a week. I noticed after a month of taking the shake my overall mood in general changed. Remember I told you I was a very tired, cranky, and moody individual. I was so overweight my body had absolutely no energy whatsoever. When your body has no energy it pretty much ruins everything. You don't want to do anything. I can say that this shake had a profound effect on that mindset, and was a key ingredient in making <u>The Jump Rope Diet</u> much more effective. I made sure that I didn't add any sugar to the mix. I also made sure to put cinnamon in my oatmeal. The cinnamon had a profound effect on my health as well. Remember cinnamon is nothing but pure fiber, and fiber is incredibly important to the digestive system. As long as you're going to the bathroom often you're losing weight. You want to make sure you're getting as much fiber as you possibly can. That's why I added apples to the mix because apples are rich in fiber. It's also why I added blueberries to the mix because they're rich in fiber as well. I wanted to make sure that I upped my fiber intake by as much as I possibly could. I also wanted to make sure I was getting a ton of vitamin C.

Vitamin C is the reason why I made sure to add a whole orange. I added bananas to the mix because I wanted to make sure that I was getting a lot of potassium. Bananas are good for Vitamin B6. Vitamin B6 is something that you'll see in almost every natural energy supplement.

Cranberries were just another source of fiber. They have even more fiber than blueberries. They're also packed full of antioxidants. The strawberries were mostly for flavor at first until I started doing more research, and I realize that strawberries were amazing. They can help prevent heart disease, stroke, cancer, high blood pressure, constipation, allergies, asthma diabetes, and depression. Strawberries are ah incredibly effective antioxidant.

Oatmeal is packed full of iron it's probably one of the most iron rich foods out there. It also has an extremely large amount of vitamin B6, magnesium, and vitamin A not to mention 6 grams of protein. Speaking of protein maybe I should discuss what I had for lunch.

Everyday for lunch I would have grilled chicken, beans, and a protein shake. My lunch was all about protein intake. For lunch I wanted to make sure I was getting as much protein in my body as possible. That's why I made sure I had grilled chicken because chicken has an extremely large amount of protein. Chicken is one of the most protein rich meats on the planet, and it's healthier for you than beef or pork. Not to mention it's a lot easier to cook especially if you know how to bake. It's even easier if you have a griller like one of those commercial grillers that drain out all the grease. Everyday when I woke up in the morning I would turn on my rice cooker, and add one cup or two cups of black beans. I chose black beans because they're low in calories. One cup is only 624 calories, and because they are extremely high in dietary fiber, you get 29 grams in one cup. Also because they're high in protein you get 39 grams of protein in one cup. They have an extremely large amount of iron, and ah extremely large amount of magnesium, and calcium so it was an obvious choice. Black beans are ah incredibly healthy super food with 2760 mg of potassium.

The body is supposed to consume at least 30 to 38 grams of fiber every day if you're a man. If you're a woman it's about 25 grams of fiber everyday. So basically one cup of black beans would almost be enough fiber for the day for a man and more than enough for a woman. If you read up on black beans you'll understand just how nutritious they really are. It's one of the most underestimated super foods on the planet. The only substitute that I would ever use for black beans if I didn't have them is quinoa. Quinoa is probably the greatest food on the planet, and the only food that has pretty much all the amino acids that you need. I also made sure that I had a whey protein isolate shake everyday.

For dinner I ate pretty much anything I wanted. I just made sure that I didn't eat any fast food. I completely cut out fast food in general. For dinner I would have a meal with black beans on the side. I would have ground turkey meat, chicken, or fish. I wouldn't have any beef or pork. So I would have some turkey tacos with black beans, and cheese, or I would have some turkey nachos with black beans, and cheese. Sometimes I would eat some salmon, beans, and rice. As long as I added the black beans to the meal I would create any combination I wanted. Eating beans with your meal helps the digestive process. It increases the nutritional value of the meal. I didn't really eat any dessert, but I've never been one to eat dessert anyway so it wasn't a big change for me.

My diet wasn't too extreme it wasn't anything that was impractical. All my food was good it wasn't like I had to eat nasty stuff that I didn't like. When you have to eat a bunch of nasty stuff that you don't like eventually you're going to give up on it. I loved the food I was eating! My shake was delicious, and my oatmeal was always good especially with cinnamon. I never put sugar in my oatmeal I just added cinnamon to it. If I wanted it to taste good I would add some honey. I made sure that I got my honey from the whole food store. Black beans are my favorite especially once you season them with some Lawry's, and some pepper. The grilled chicken was always good because I mean grilled chicken is awesome. Sometimes I would grill chicken and have a chicken black bean salad. It tasted great! My diet gave me energy, power, and change my mood all together. It's the main reason why I was able to go on. If I never changed my diet I would have never saw any positive effects from <u>The Jump Rope Diet</u> in the first place because I wouldn't be able to do it. My intention was never to change my diet for weight loss, but to promote energy production. I simply wanted to feel better, and run longer, and this diet accomplished that for me. I didn't find it difficult. If you can find food that has similar nutritious value that you actually find delicious by all means go about it in your own way. I'm just telling you exactly what I did. I don't want to leave any details out because that might be the one detail that contributed to my progression. If you choose to follow my diet to the letter it is more likely that you will see the same results that I did. Maybe you might find some loopholes that I didn't find. You might be able to improve upon the diet. If so please don't hoard information comment, and add your perspective. Tell the people of the dietary changes you implement that worked in combination with The Jump Rope Diet. Maybe tells us some of the vitamins that you used in combination with The Jump Rope Diet. Share other forms of jump rope training you've tried in combination with The Jump Rope Diet that worked for you.

Wrap Up

I have started many fitness programs, and gave up. The only fitness programs that I've ever finished are The Jump Rope Diet, The Kettlebell Cleanse, and The Sprint Diet. That's because these programs work they're clear, and easy to understand. <u>The Jump Rope Diet</u> is clear-cut, and dry. It gave me back my health my energy an my life. I hope that you will find the same success with it. I hope that you will stick to the program regardless of whatever life throws your way. Remember motivation is the number one key to continuing results. You're going to feel amazing you're going to look amazing, and you're going to have a better attitude towards life.

When you take fitness, and health seriously you achieve ah positive mindset. If you feel good you'll think more positively. If you feel bad you'll think negatively. It's all about your default setting. Individuals that are healthy are usually at a positive default setting. Individuals that are not healthy are usually at a negative default setting. Optimism is a great key to life. Children are very optimistic that's why they're always in a great mood. Children believe things are going to get better every single day. That optimism seems to leave us, as we become adults. We are no surer about tomorrow than we are about today.

Adults look at 5 years down the line, and think maybe things will be better. We don't look at tomorrow, and think tomorrow is going to be the greatest day of my life. That's the level of optimism you need to get from point A to point B. You have to believe that what you're doing is working. If you stop believing in the process most likely you won't continue it. The jump rope diet will set you on a great path toward a healthy life. Respect your body, and nurture your mind. Remember what you eat is just as important as how much you exercise. Be cautious of the foods that you put into your body. As long as you lower your calorie intake by 500 you should be just fine.

First you need to understand how many calories your body needs to operate. You can find that information on many websites. Just give them your height, weight, and age than click away. If you are a 200 pound six foot two male you need about 2600 calories to maintain your current weight. To lose weight you would lower your calorie consumption to 2100. Combined with the calories that you lose with the jump rope diet you can expect great results. With that I bid you farewell. Have a happy, and healthy life from the Workout King.

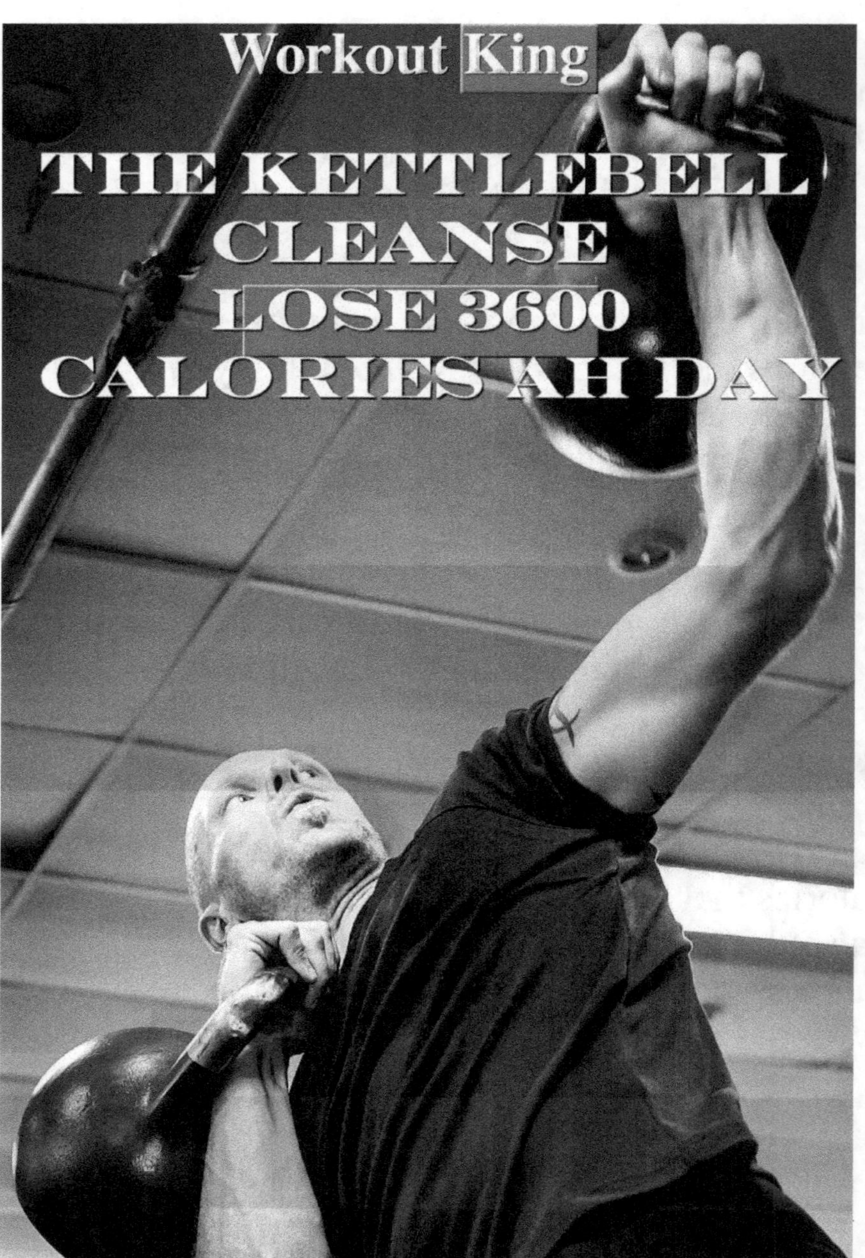

Workout King
THE KETTLEBELL
CLEANSE
LOSE 3600
CALORIES AH DAY

The Kettlebell Cleanse

My Story

If you're looking for a book with perfect spelling, and punctuation than you've come to the wrong place. If you're looking for a book with accurate, and useful information than you've come to the right place.

When I discovered the Kettlebell I was going through a hard time. I had no idea what I was doing. No form of exercise was working for me. I didn't want to go to the gym because I was ashamed of the way I looked. I wanted to do a workout that would preserve my muscle, but would help me lose fat. I started doing research, and by the grace of good luck I ran into the Kettlebell. At first I had no idea what it was or how it worked. I just knew that it was something that I'd seen before in the stores, but I never actually picked it up. I didn't know it came in different sizes. I didn't know what size I needed. All I know is when I started using it my body started to change. At first I didn't know any of the routines or moves. I had no idea you could work out your entire body with it! Little by little I learn different moves, and which muscles they targeted. Little by little I started to discover different combinations of moves that helped me lose weight quickly, and efficiently. Having a kettlebell is like having a gym in your house. People say that the Kettlebell builds muscle, but that depends on how often you up the weight. You have to increase the resistance if you want to increase your muscle size. If you start off with ah 10-pound kettlebell you want to up the weight to 15 or 20. You work towards 30 than you work towards 40, and so on. Don't use a ten-pound kettlebell for three months that's the last thing you want to do! You're not going to see the results you're looking for if you do that. I continued to increase the weight. I continued to increase the complexity of my workouts, and my results shine through.

Throughout my weight-loss journey I would pick things up, and put them down immediately. I didn't feel like anything was working. The Kettlebell is different. For some reason I like doing it. I could feel that it was working for me. I could feel that it was having a positive effect on my body. It wasn't just helping me lose weight it was helping me gain muscle. I could feel muscle growing in me every time I worked out. Above all the kettlebell builds muscle endurance.

I've always had a fear of putting in limitless amounts of work to get no results. It seems like that was always the case with the majority of the workouts I tried. With the Kettlebell what I put in was what I got out that's why I respect it.

The Benefits Of Kettlebell Training

The Kettlebell combines cardio with strength training. I mean drop the mic on stage that's pretty much the greatest benefit of all time. There are very few exercises I can name that actually combine cardio with strength training. Sprinting has the same effect, and guess who has a book on that this guy. It's called The Sprint Diet check it out it's a great read. When you combine cardio, and strength training you get high calorie loss without loss of muscle. Ah hour of kettlebell training can burn 1200 calories that's a lot of calories. Compare that to 500 calories for an hour on the treadmill there's no competition. The Kettlebell wins hands down! You would have to do almost two, and ah half hours worth of work just to match one hour of kettlebell training. That's not even considering the internal benefits that Kettlebell training has over the treadmill. Even if you consider a more calories aggressive machine like the elliptical you're still only going to get eight maybe 900 calories for an hour. Still no match for the Kettlebell! Not only are you going to burn more calories by using the Kettlebell, but you're also going to build muscle. You're not going to build any muscle on treadmills! It doesn't matter if we're talking about the bike, the elliptical, or even the stair climber the kettlebell's going to win every single time it has no equal. The kettlebell is not nearly as hard as some people make it seem. If you start off slow, and learn the essential exercises it's not hard at all. If anything it can be fun once you become proficient. You want to start off with three basic moves. Once you master them you do more complicated movements. You just need to build up some strength, and some coordination first.

Beginners Moves And Kettlebell Selection

You have to be careful when choosing a kettlebell. You don't want to pick anything that's too heavy. If you do you might throw your back out. This is why it's best to pick your kettlebell in the store. It's easier to shop for a kettlebell online once you've already had some experience with a real kettlebell. Go into the store, and try some moves with some of the kettlebells. See if it feels right. As long as it's not to light it's the right size. If you're a female I suggest you start off with a 10-pound kettlebell. If you're stronger than by all means buy something more advanced. If you're a male I suggest that you start off with a 15 to 20 pound kettlebell. As you become stronger the weight we'll get lighter. At this point you want to up the weight so you can continue gaining muscle. If you keep lifting the same weight you're not going to notice a difference no matter how hard you work! Now that we got that out of the way let's talk about beginner techniques.

First up is _The Kettlebell Swing_. The kettlebell swing is the most popular kettlebell exercise. It works the hips, glutes, hamstrings, lats, ABS, shoulders, chest, and your grip. It's one of the most effective exercises you can do with the Kettlebell. I personally have seen series results from the kettlebell swing. It's my favorite kettlebell move. In the photo you can see exactly how to do a kettlebell swing. As you can see it's all about the hips. When you bring the weight back up the momentum from you thrusting your hips forward is what carries it to the top not your arms. You're thrusting with your hips while squeezing your abs, and your glutes simultaneously. Just make sure you don't let go of the Kettlebell. I did that once and boy did I cause some damage. This exercise makes you so much better at all the other kettlebell moves. It strengthens the key muscles you need to perform more advanced movements.

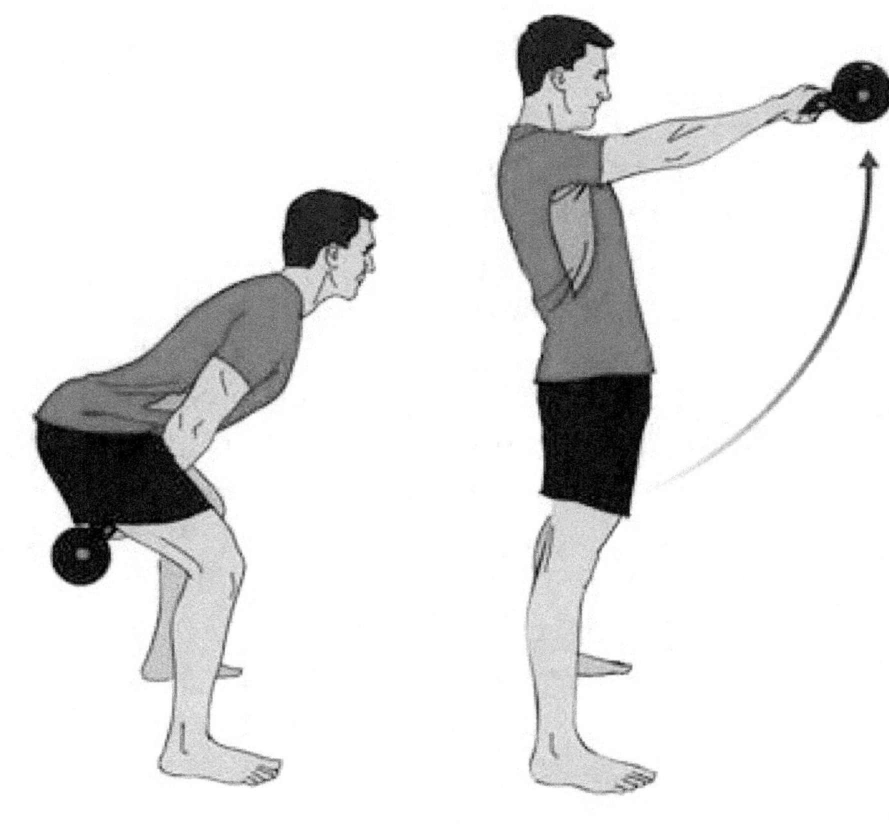

The second move is _The Around The Body Pass_. The around the body pass is the most basic kettlebell move there it's. It's one of the most important moves because it strengthens the core, and the obliques. The kettlebell is a core-blasting beast. Almost every single exercise requires you use your core in some way. The around the body pass strengthens the core, and your oblique's preparing your body to deal with advanced compound movements. The more advanced the move the more it will require core stability. Even though this move looks simple at first you might drop the Kettlebell, I know I did. Passing a heavy weight behind your back might be a little more difficult than you think. Passing the weight behind you forces your core to stabilize your body that's what makes it a key core workout.

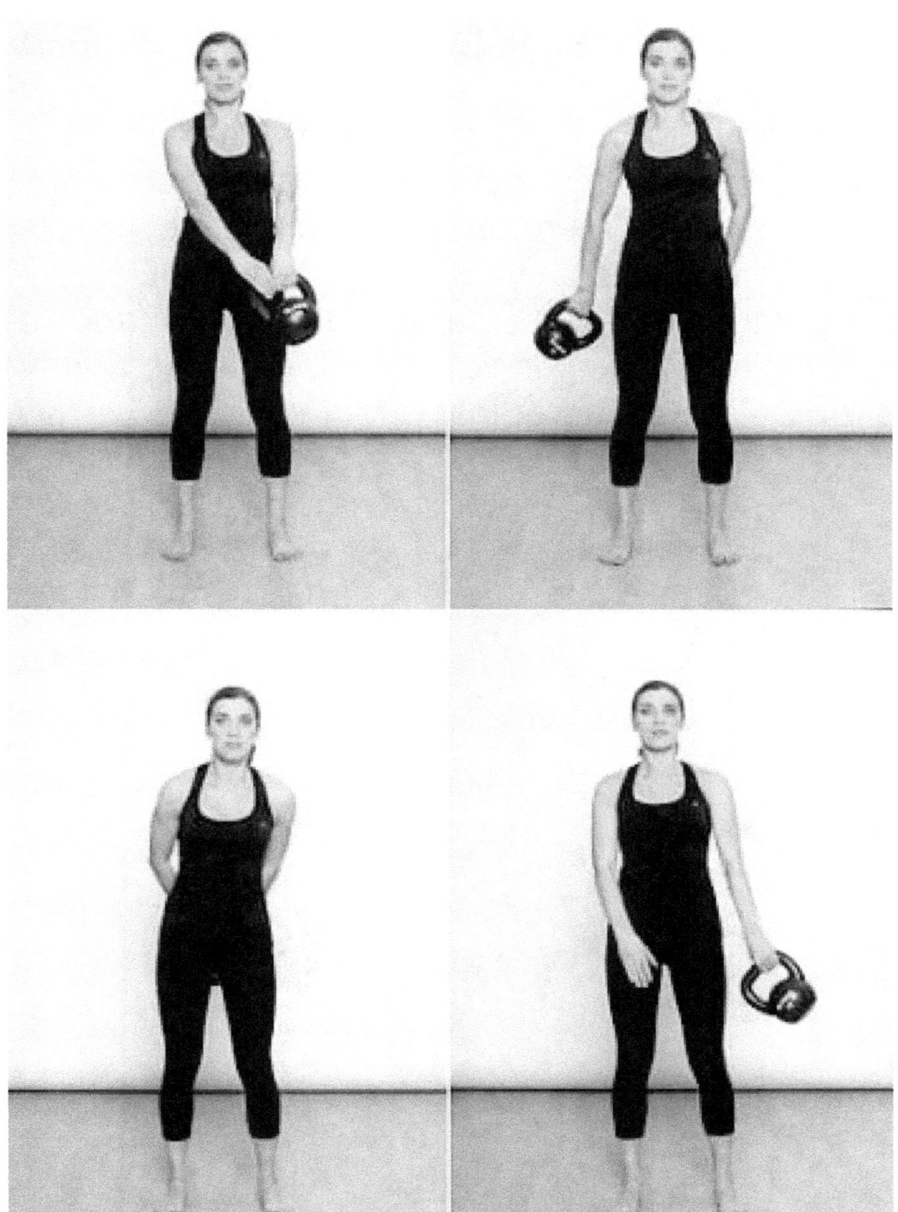

Number three is the _Two Hand Overhead Press_. _The Two Hand Overhead Press_ is a very key beginner moves. It works the shoulders, back, chest, triceps, and the core. These are key muscles that you're going to need throughout any kettlebell routine. Below is a picture of how to perform the _Two Hand Overhead Press_. As you can see it's incredibly simple yet it is incredibly effective.

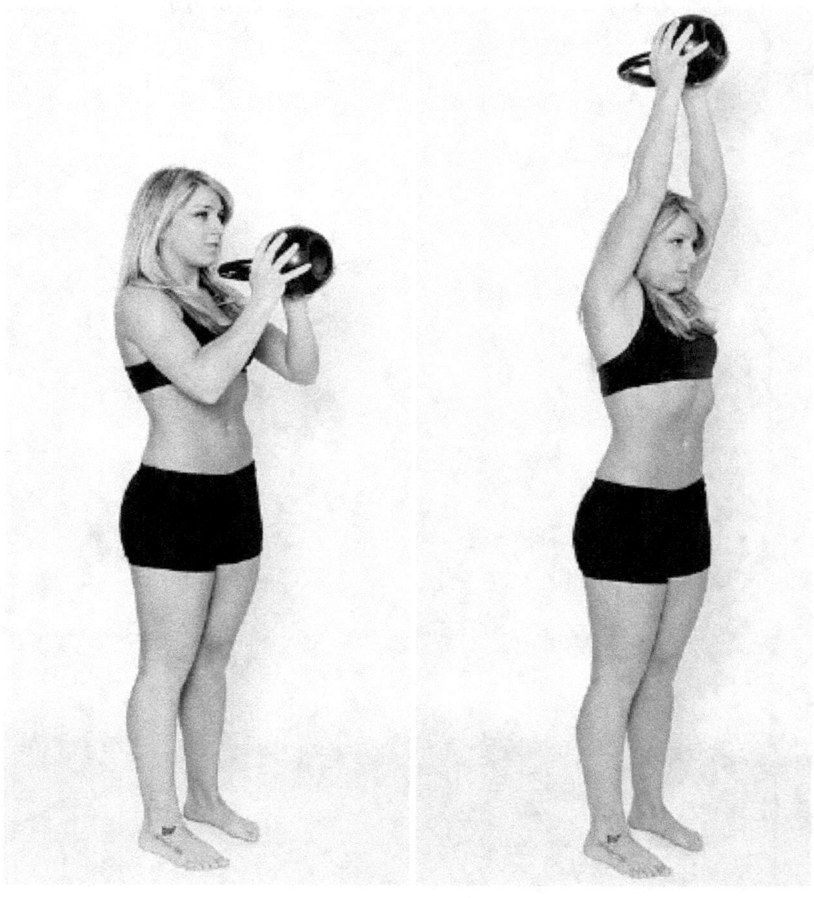

As a beginner workout you would combine all three of these exercises together. You want to do this for a period of at least 30 minutes. A good combination would be 10 minutes of each individual exercise. If that's too boring for you than simply do five minutes of all three two times. Do 30 minutes a day for 15 days, and I guarantee you will notice a difference. In those 15 days you'll build up enough strength, and endurance to take on more intermediate movements.

Intermediate Training

When beginning intermediate training it is best to up the weight. If you want continuous results you must increase the difficulty to make sure that you continue gaining muscle.

The first on the list is _The Kettlebell Sit Up_. _The Kettlebell Sit Up_ is a very effective technique. It's a weighted abdominal exercise. People forget that abs are just like any muscle, using body weight alone won't be enough to make them pop out. If you want ab definition you have to increase the weight resistance. The Kettlebell is a great way of doing just that.

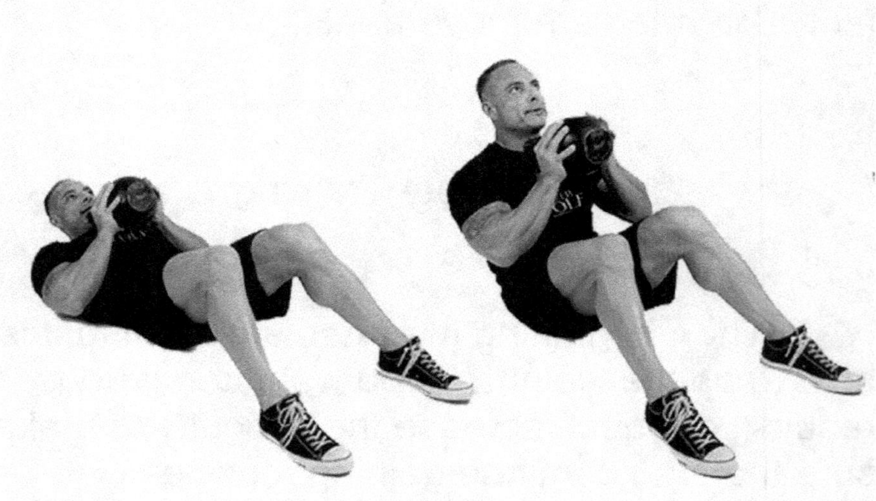

The next exercise is _The Russian Twist_. _The Russian Twist_ is a classic kettlebell move. It's incredibly effective at working the obliques. If you don't want those pesky love handles _The Russian Twists_ is the exercise for you. Take a look at the way she's holding the Kettlebell. As you can see she's keeping her back stable making sure not to lose control.

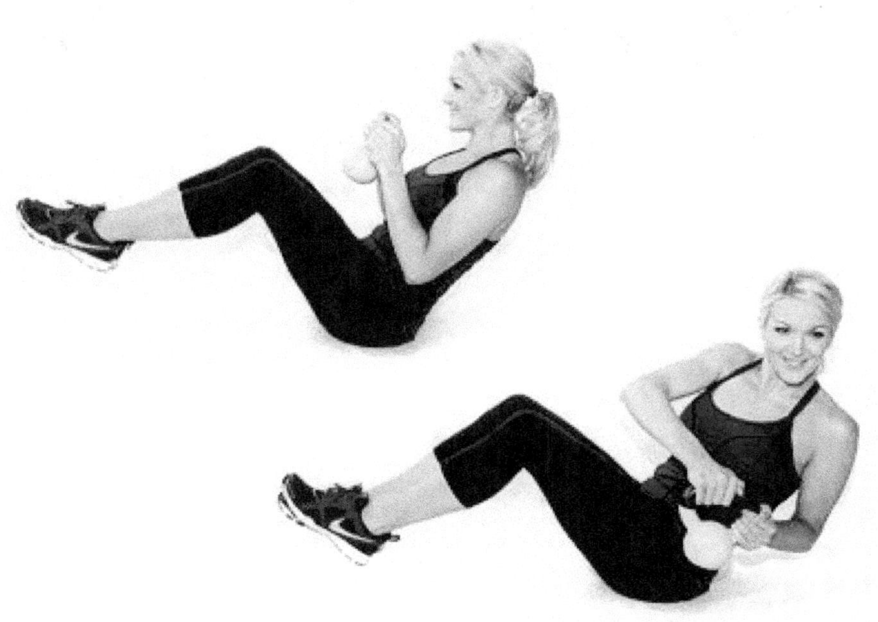

Next on the list is _The Figure Eight_. This is another exercise that's incredibly effective at working your abdominals. It also has the added benefit of working your hamstrings. Always keep your back straight so that you don't bend forward when you passed the Kettlebell between your legs.

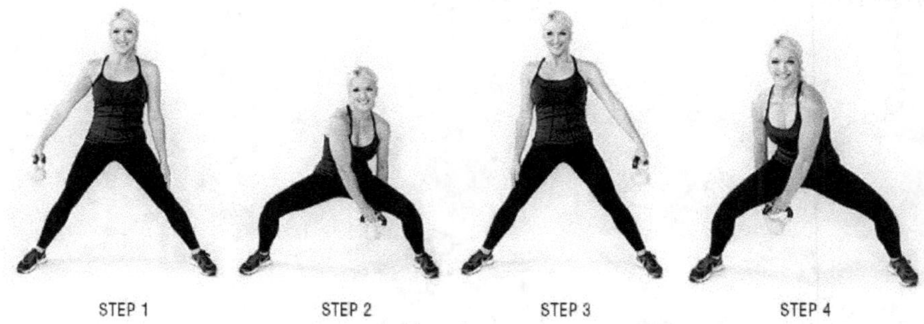

Next on the list is _The Two Handed Squat_. _The Two Handed Squat_ works the quadriceps, hamstrings, gluteus maximus, and erector spinae. It's a very simple move when you look at it, but with repetition your quads will start to burn.

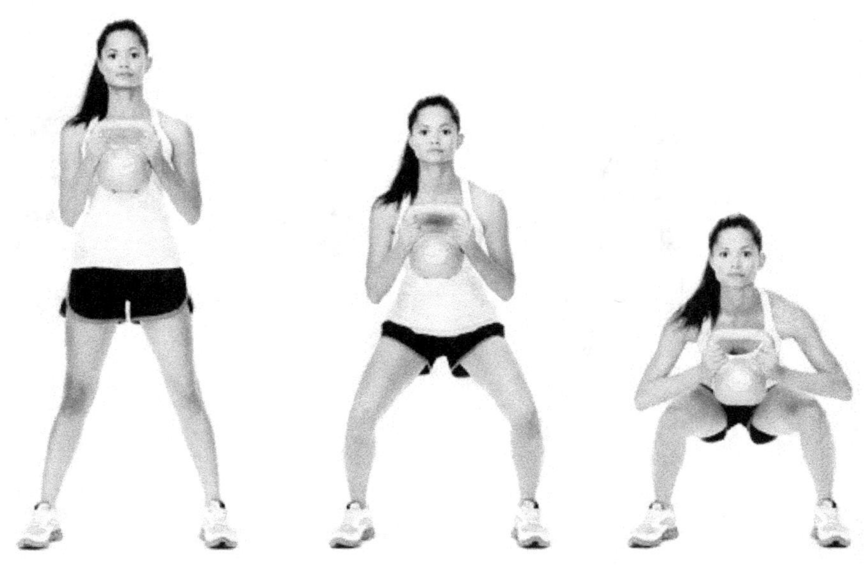

Next would be <u>*The Squat & Press*</u>. *The Squat & Press* is one of my favorite moves. It works the majority of the body. Glutes, hamstrings, quadriceps, core, back, and arms. It's a very simple compound movement, but it's incredibly effective.

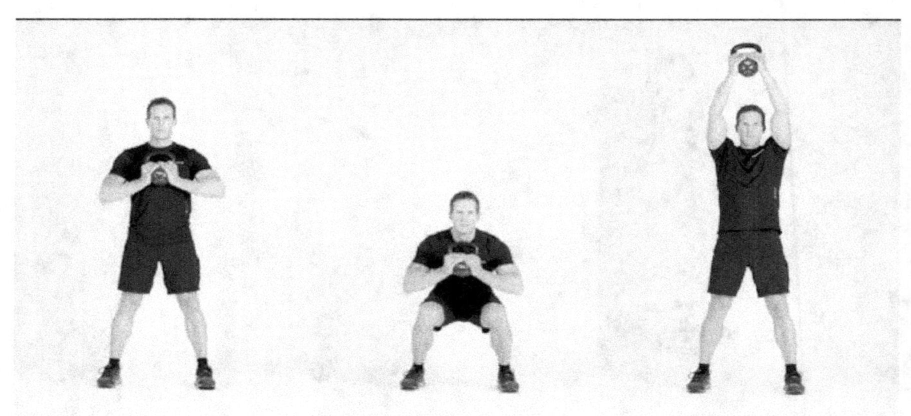

The next move is _The Clean_. The Clean works the majority of the body. You get to work your chest, your shoulders, your back, your biceps, triceps, your abs, legs, and glutes all in one move.

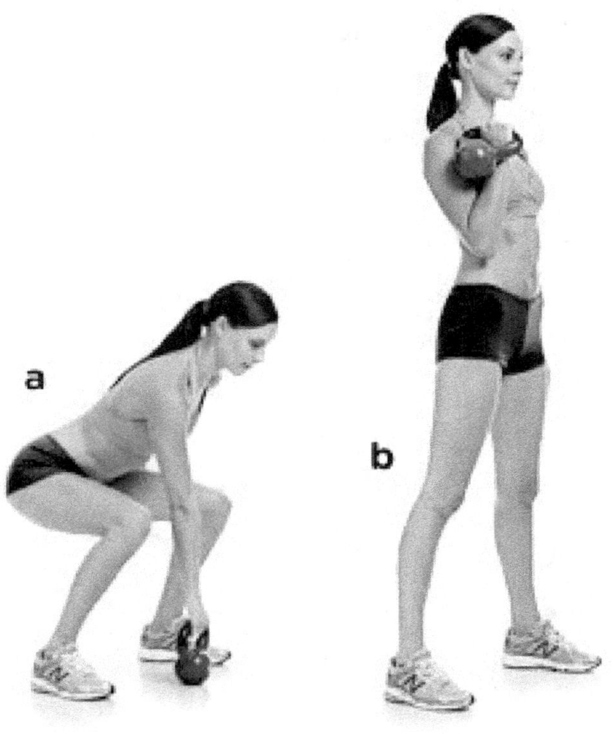

Next on the list is _The Snatch_. Now I know the name sounds a little funny, but the workout is actually incredibly effective. _The Snatch_ works the hamstrings, quads, back, and shoulders. If you're looking to create stability in your body increasing your balance, and control the snatch is a good move to practice. If you look at the photo below you can see that the move is all about momentum.

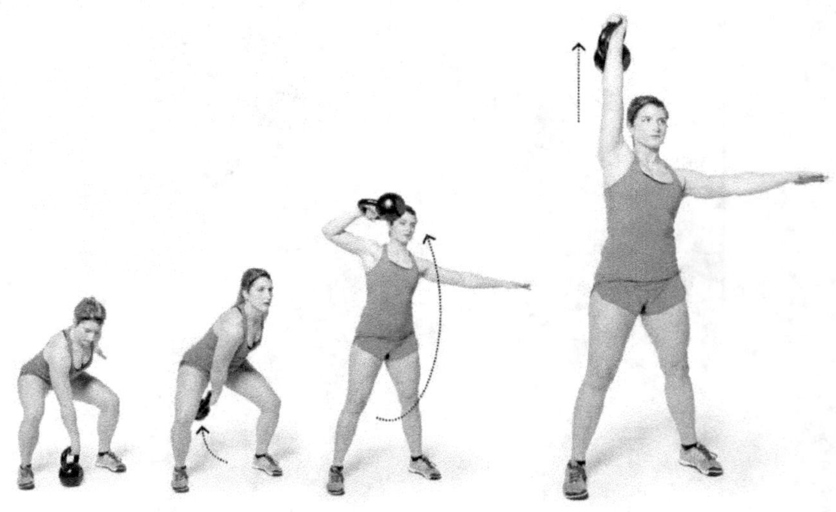

Next on the list is _The Lunge Row_. The Lunge Row is good for your rear shoulders, glutes, quads, side shoulders, triceps, biceps, hamstrings, lower back, and rhomboids. Just make sure to keep your back in a stable position, and pull your elbow as far back as you can. If you're looking to create extra strength in your back this is definitely one of the better kettlebell moves.

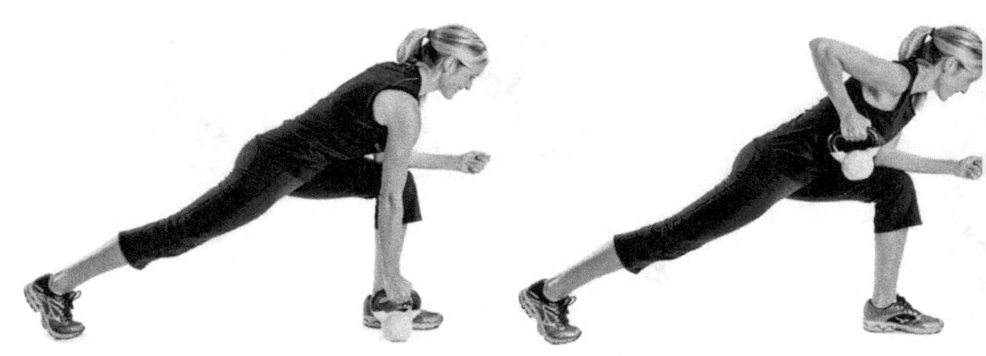

Next is _The Kettlebell One Arm Row_. _The One Arm Row_ works the rear deltoids, trappe middle region, lats, and lower back. It's an incredibly effective yet incredibly simple movement. You just want to make sure you don't jerk the weight. Lift in a fluid, and controlled motion.

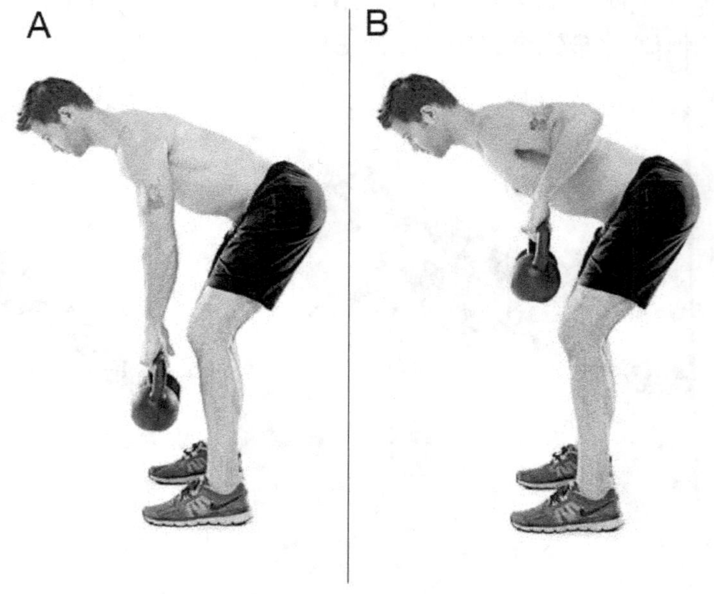

Next on the list is _The Lunge Press_. _The Lunge Press_ is good for your thighs, core, and back. If you're looking for a strong intermediate workout to increase your leg strength this is the work out for you.

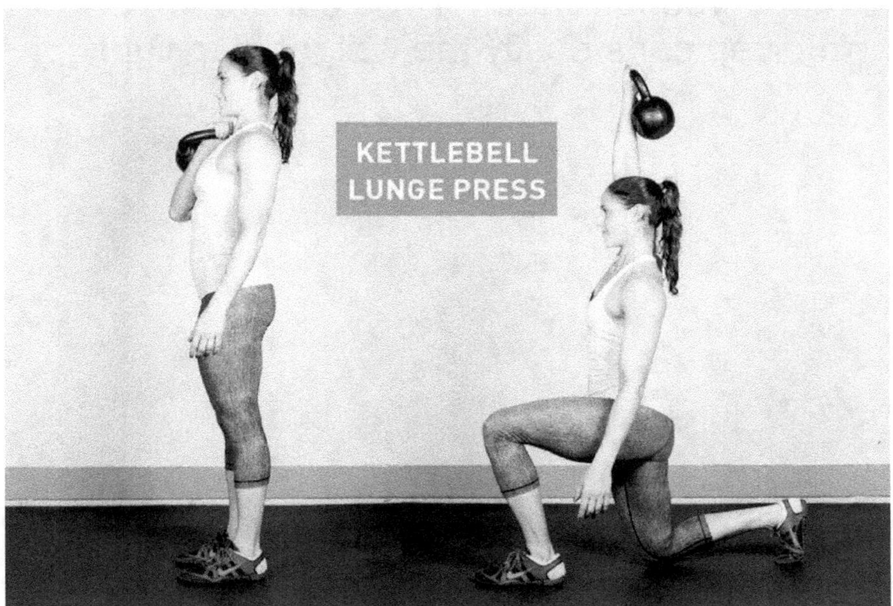

.

Next on our list is <u>*The Bicep Curl*</u>. As you probably already know *The Bicep Curl* works the biceps. Try a one-arm bicep curl. You can grip the Kettlebell by the horns, and do a two arm bicep curl. The Bicep Curl is a good way to judge your strength. If you can do ten one arm bicep curls easily the weight is to light.

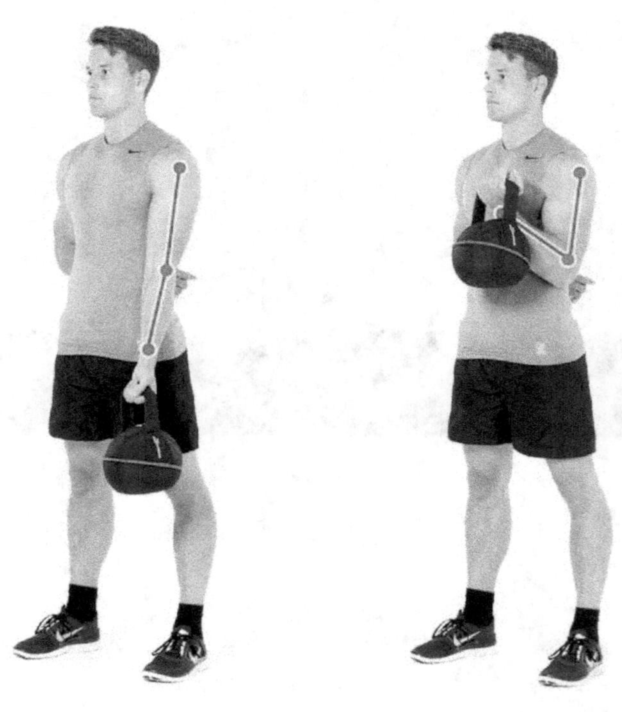

Next on our list is the rotating lunge. The rotating lunge works the obliques, ABS, quads, glutes, and hamstrings. The Move may look simple, but trust me balance is a key factor. When doing *The Rotating Lunge* you have to stabilize your core, back, and legs. It's a full-body stabilization workout making it great for stability, and balance enhancement. If you can do a set of these with out wobbling, my hat goes off to you.

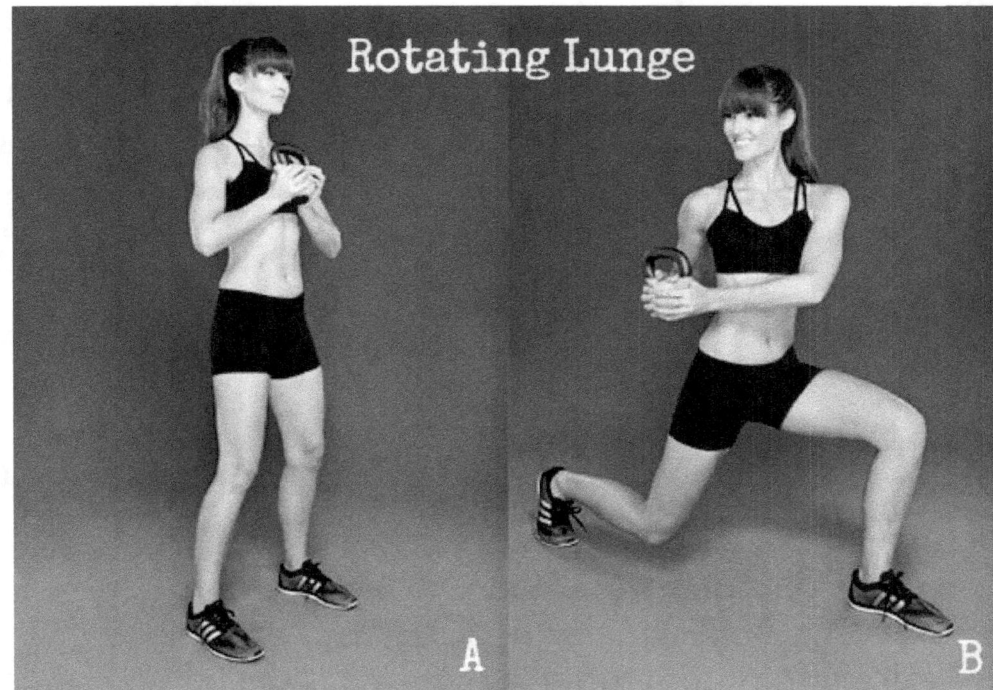

Last but not least is *The Sumo Squat Lift.* Also called *The Sumo Squat High Pull*. *The Sumo Squat Lift* works the quads, glutes, hamstrings, biceps, and upper back. It's one of those incredible compound movements targeting a large range of muscles.

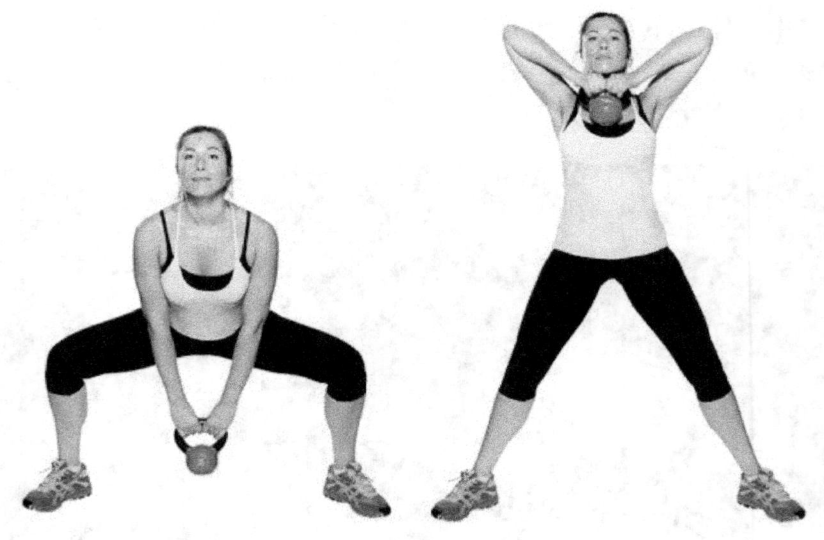

You can mix, and match these moves together in any combination. Within a 36-minute session you can do 2 minutes of each one of these workouts. These intermediate workouts will increase your core stability allowing you a greater range of motion. They will also increase your flexibility, and muscle endurance. Do 36 minutes a day for 30 days. In 30 days you should be ready to move on.

You're going to have more energy than you've ever had before.

Advance Training

Now that you're on an advanced level you may be thinking of upping the weight considerably. Be careful you want to make sure that you can handle the weight. If you get a kettlebell that's too heavy you might not be able to do some of the exercises in the advanced program. Therefore it might be best for you to only go up by 5 or 10 pounds at first. When you get the hang of the movements, and increase your strength you can increase the weight considerably.

The first move is <u>*The Half Get Up*</u>. *The Half Get Up* is a very advanced move. It will require stability, and strength beyond any other move you've done so far. *The Half Get Up* works the interior deltoid, erector spinae, external obliques, gluteus maximus, internal obliques, lateral deltoid, posterior deltoid, rectus abdominis, infraspinatus, and multifarious. It's truly a powerful move. The half get up requires an extremely large amount of abdominal strength. It's one of the most effective abdominal workouts, but it's also one of the most difficult.

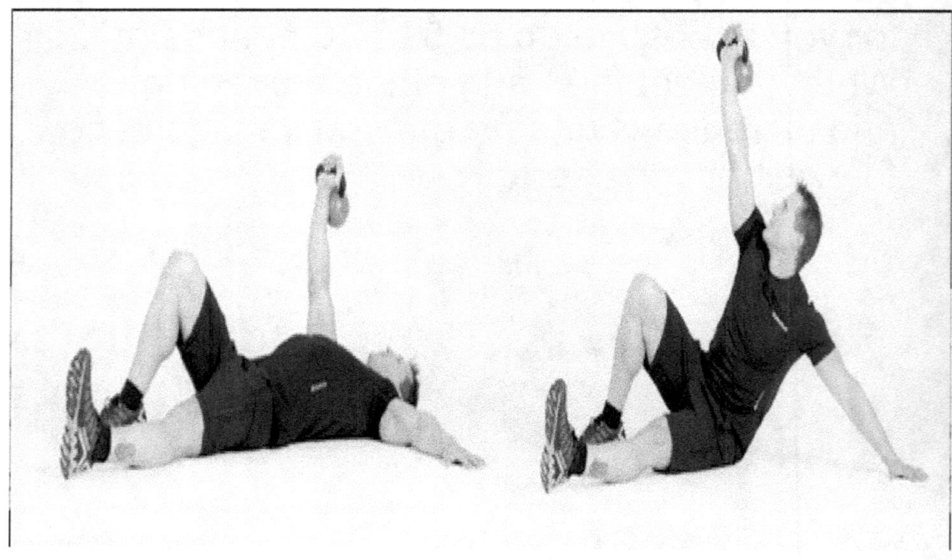

Next on the list is _The Turkish Get Up_. _The Half Get Up_ is just one piece of _The Turkish Get Up_. In my opinion _The Turkish Get Up_ is the most complex move. _The Turkish Get Up_ requires a greater range of motion, control, stability, and endurance than any other compound movement. It works every muscle that _The Half Get Up_ does including the quadriceps, traps, and hamstrings. Doing _The Turkish Get Up_ for 15 minutes is considered an advanced level workout.

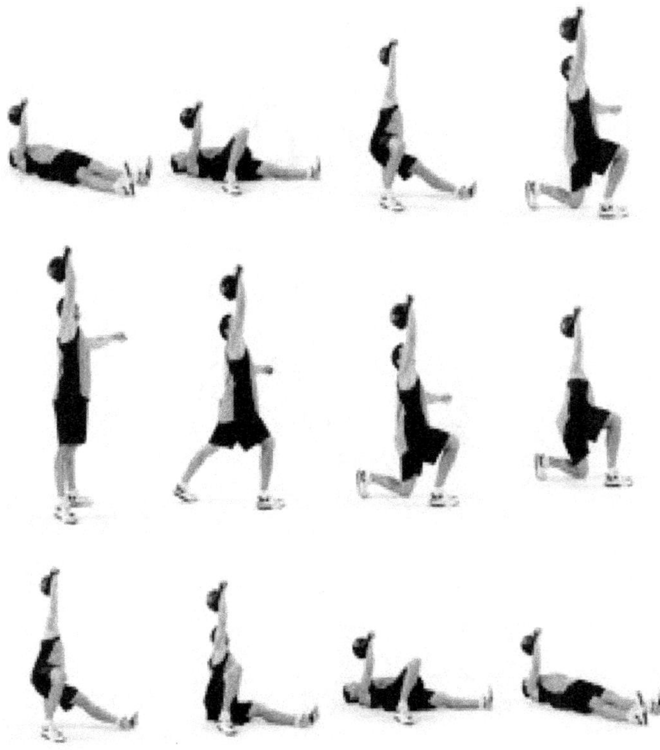

Next up is <u>*The Single Leg Deadlift*</u>. *The Single Leg Deadlift* works the latissimus dorsai, abdominals, quadriceps, and hamstrings. It's important for balance. This move creates stability, and allows you to easily balance on one leg.

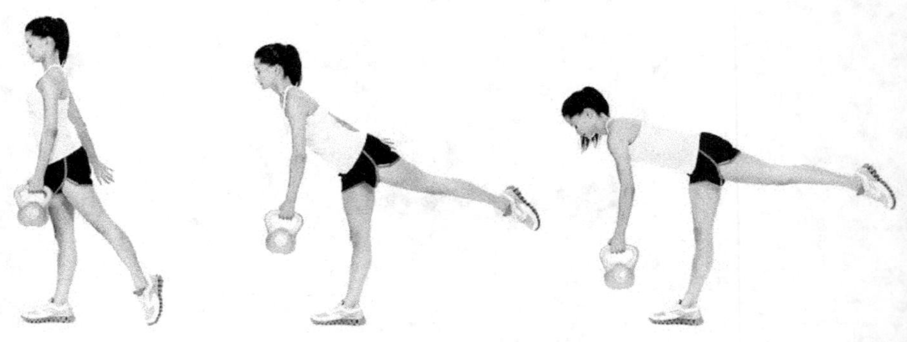

The next move is _The Overhead Jackknife_. *The Overhead Jackknife* works the triceps, and the core. It's one of those core exercises that you can easily add into your routine. Just make sure to hold on to the weight you don't want it to drop on your face.

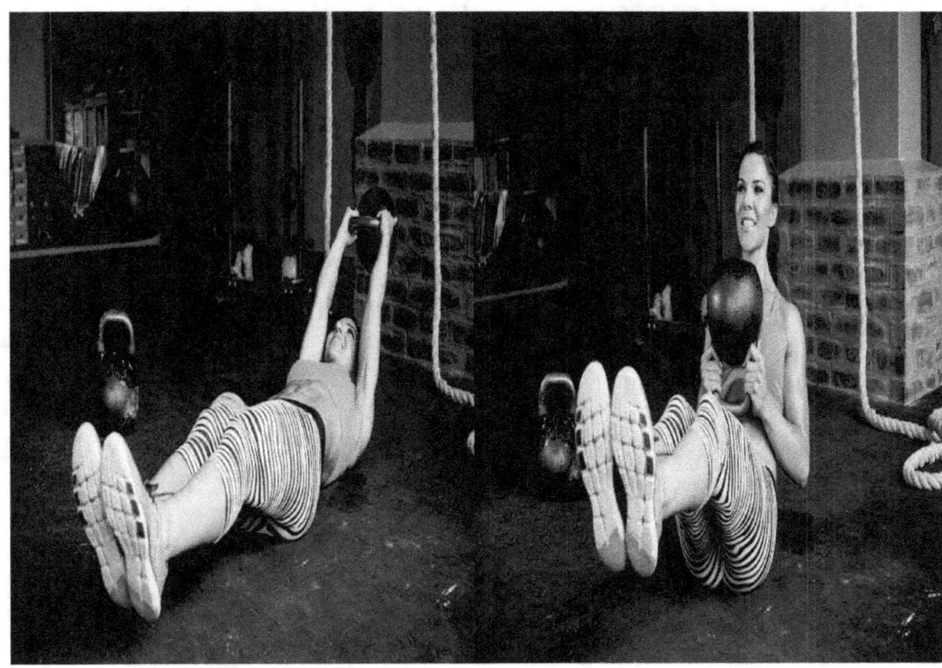

The next move is *The Chop*. *Chops* work the latissimus dorsai, abdominals, quadriceps, and gluteus maximus. To be honest chops are one of the more fun moves to do. All my friends find them quite enjoyable. Although they can be quite fun if you don't keep your balance the move could be quite dangerous near fragile objects. Make sure to keep your back straight and control the weight.

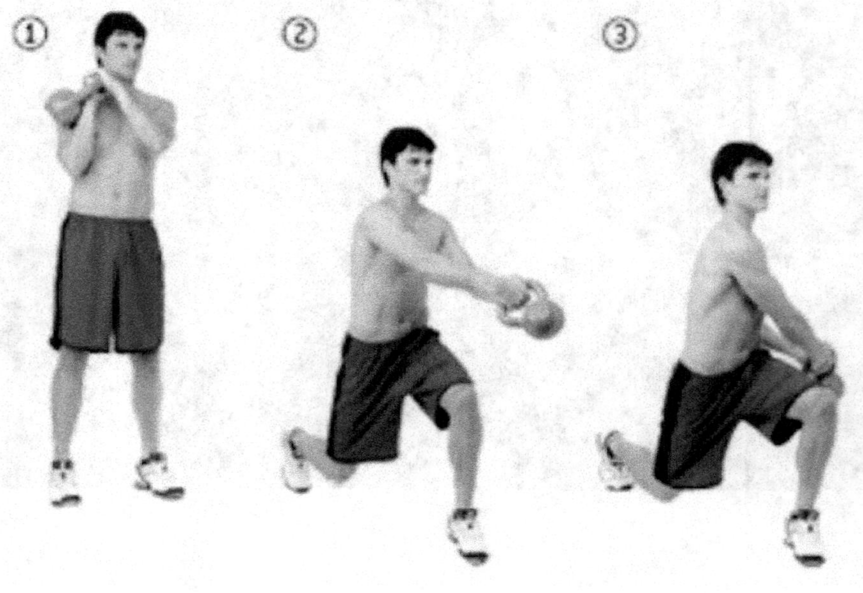

The next move is _The Clean & Press_. _The Clean & Press_ works the triceps, traps, abdominals, calves, lower back, hamstrings, and glutes. It's one of those advanced compound movements that gives you an almost full body workout. This move is guaranteed to get you ready for the summer.

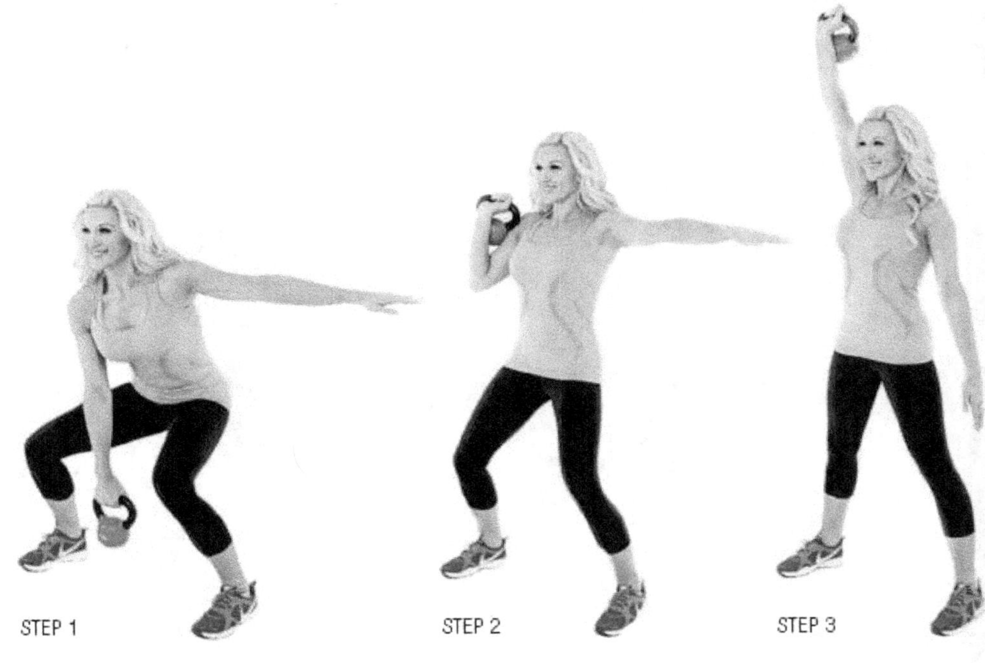

The next move is *The Two-Handed Deadlift*. This is a basic move unless you're lifting a heavy load. You have to make sure to stabilize your back otherwise you could be putting more stress on it than necessary. Remember to lift with your legs not your back or your arms. *The Two-Handed Deadlift* works the calves, quads, hamstrings, gluteus maximus, arms, core, back, trapeze, and shoulders.

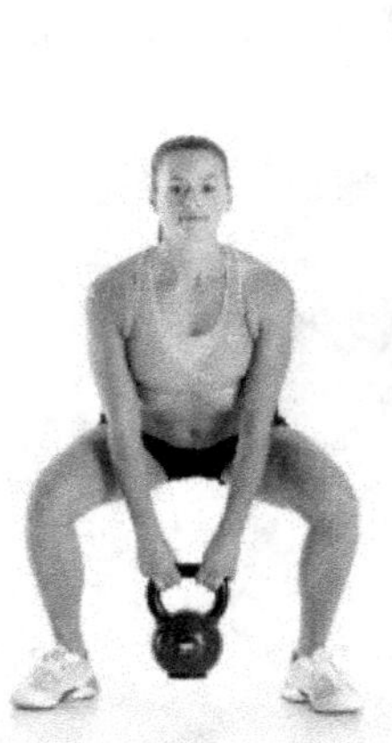
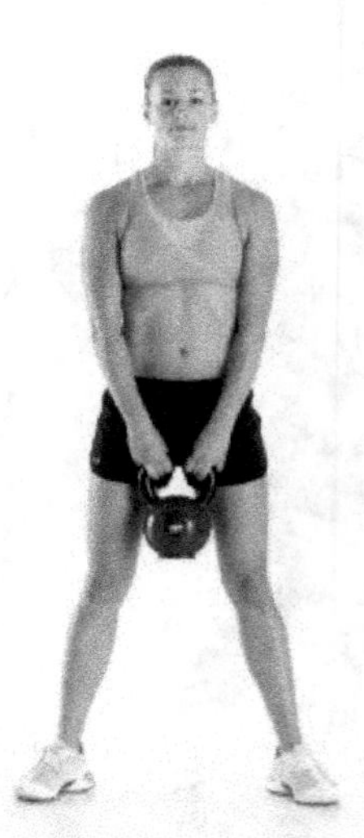

The next move is _The Windmill_. *The Windmill* increases your flexibility significantly. It also works the shoulders, hamstrings, abdominals, and the gluteus maximus.

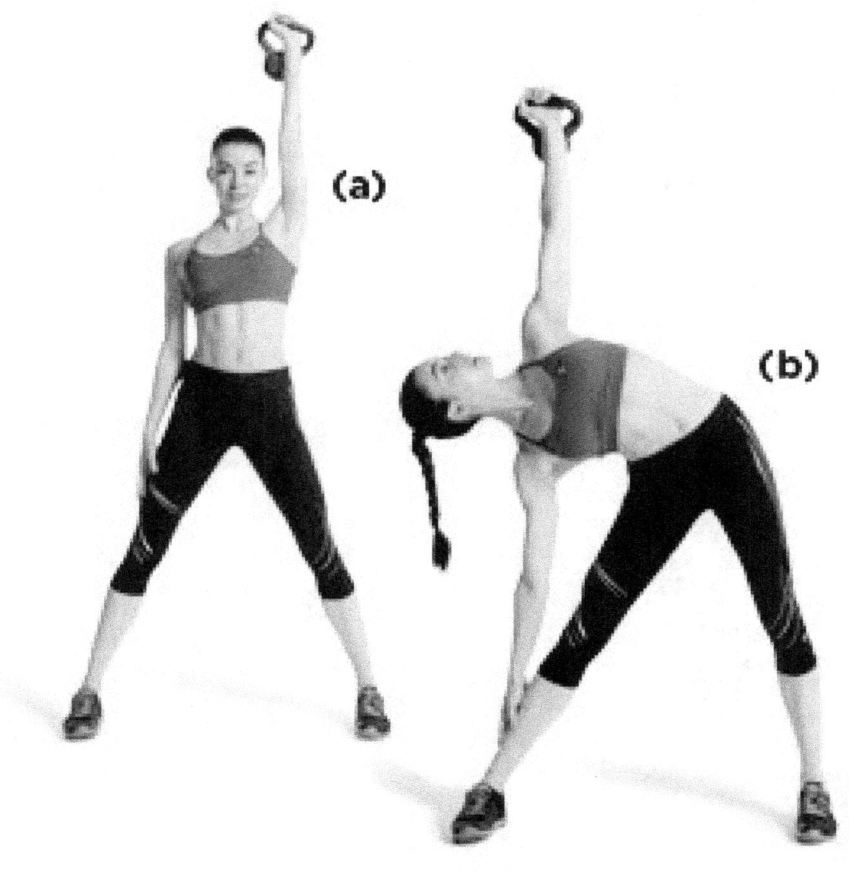

Next is *The Changing Hand Swing*. You're doing a one-arm kettlebell swing, but when you get to the top you grab the Kettlebell with your other hand. This move is very effective at strengthening your lower back, your shoulders, your gluteus maximus, your hips, hamstrings, and abdominals. *The Changing Hand Swing* is one of my go to moves. Usually if I'm in the middle of a routine, and I can't think of what to do next I just do the changing hand swing. It's truly a powerful compound workout.

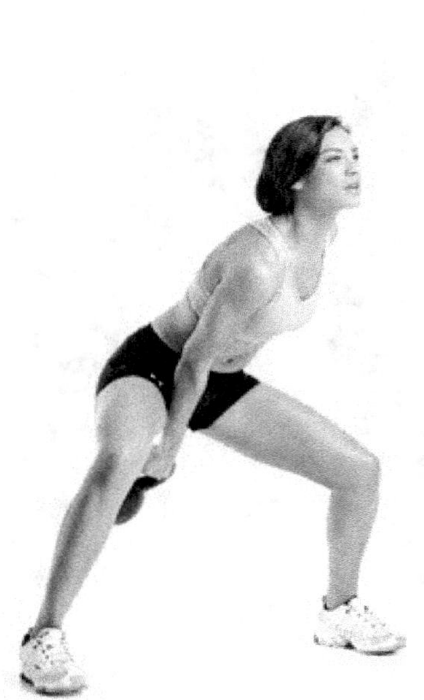
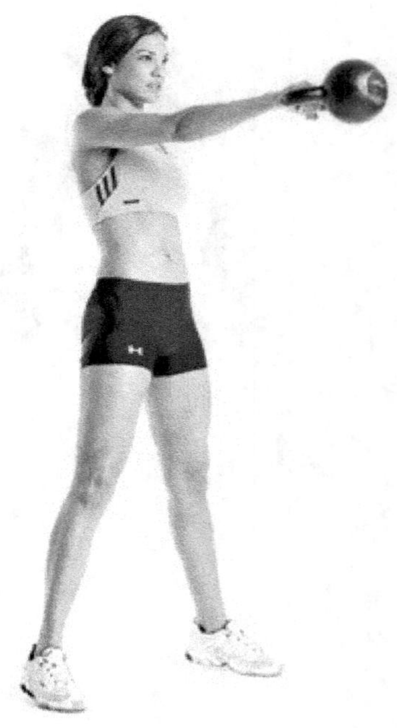

Next is _The Standing Twist._ This move is great for isolating those abdominals. You just need to make sure that you use a weight that you can control. You don't want to lean forward while you're doing the standing twist! It will cause unnecessary strain on your back.

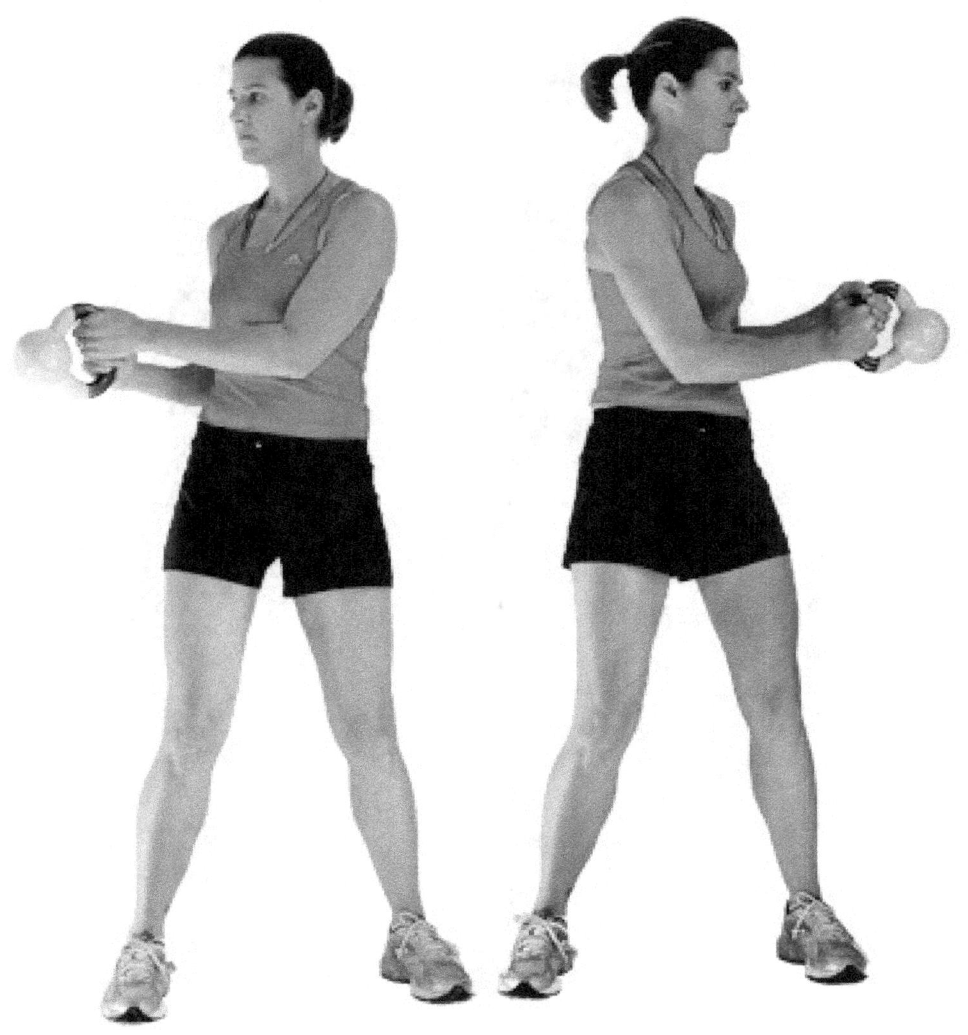

Next is *The One Arm Press*. *The One Arm Press* is looked at as a beginner move, but when doing it with heavy weight it becomes truly advanced. *The One Arm Press* works the shoulders, triceps, and core.

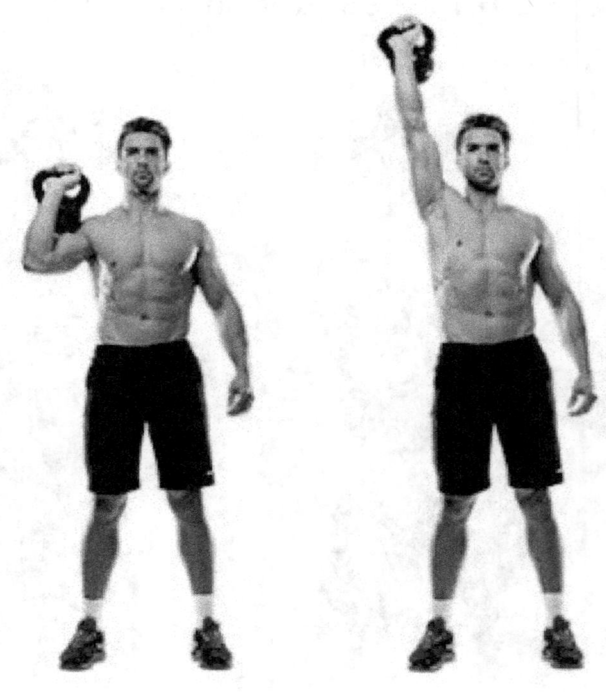

Next is _The Sit & Press_. _The Sit & Press_ works the core, and the arms. The move looks simple, but I assure you it is not. _The Sit & Press_ requires incredible core strength, and stability. You want to use a weight you can handle.

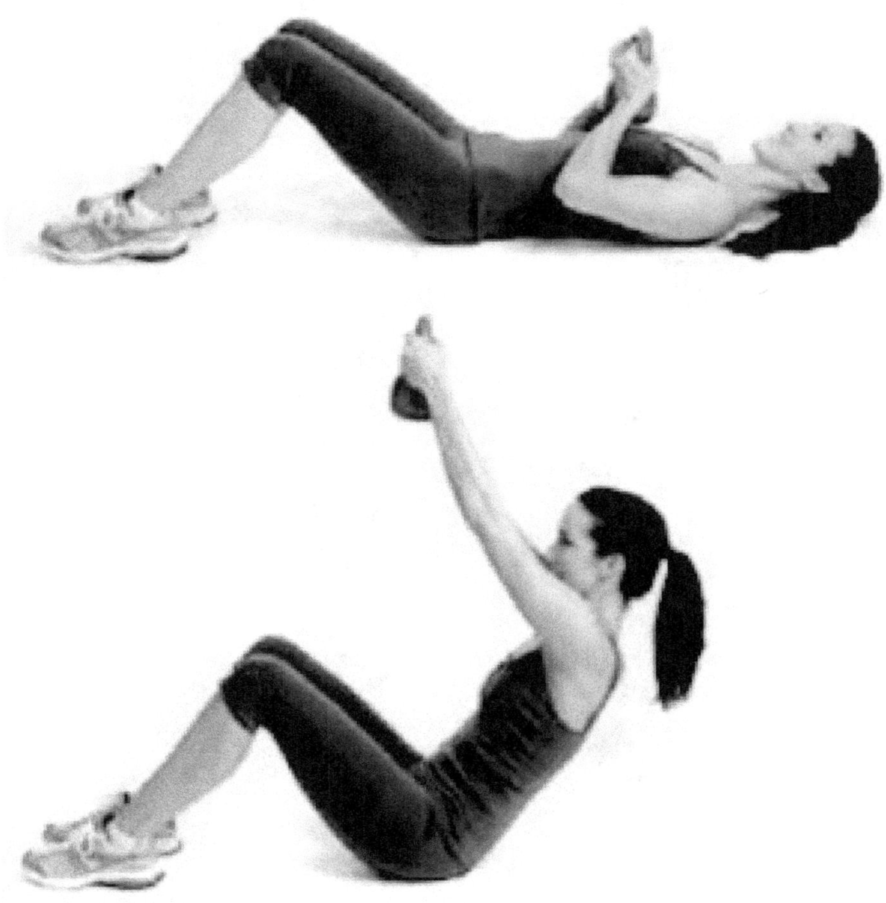

Next is <u>*The Tricep Extension*</u>. *The Tricep Extension* of course works the triceps. Depending on the weight it could be a very strenuous exercise. Make sure you hold on to the weight tightly you don't want to drop it on your head. Use your core to stabilize your body so that the weight doesn't move you backwards.

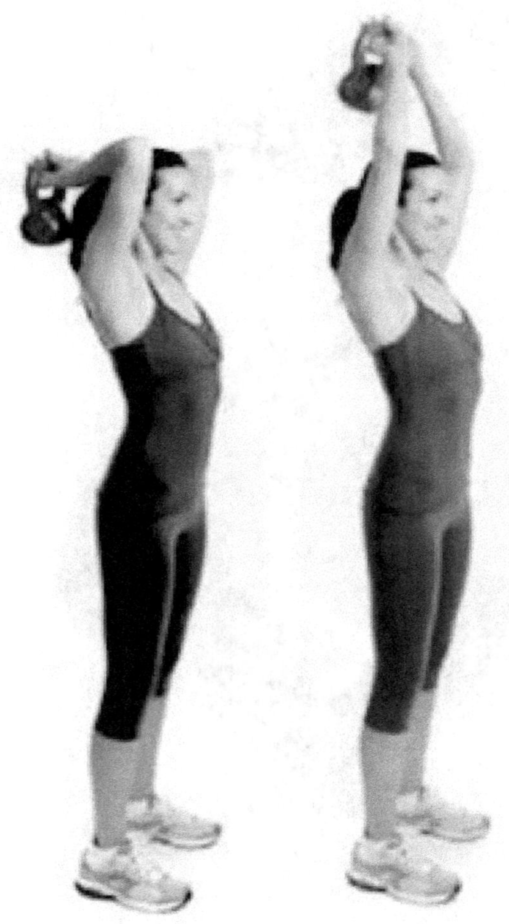

Next is _The Halo_. _The Halo_ is one of my favorite kettlebell moves. It works the deltiods, the shoulders, the pecs, the chest, the triceps, and the abdominals. Looking at the move your probably thinking how could such a simple movement work so many muscles. Well this move isn't simple at all. Keeping control of a heavy kettlebell while twisting it around your head isn't a cakewalk. In my experience this really increases your core strength, and balance.

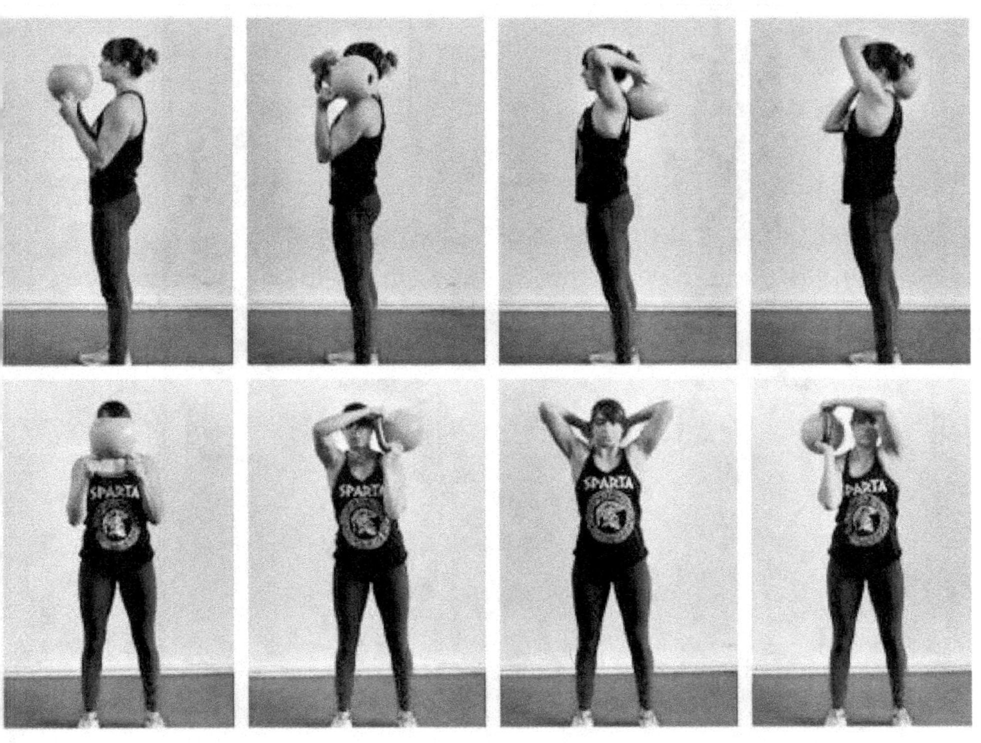

Next is _The Racked Squat_. Of course you would switch arms, and do this move on both sides. It works the quadriceps, the hamstrings, the gluteus maximus, and erector spinae.

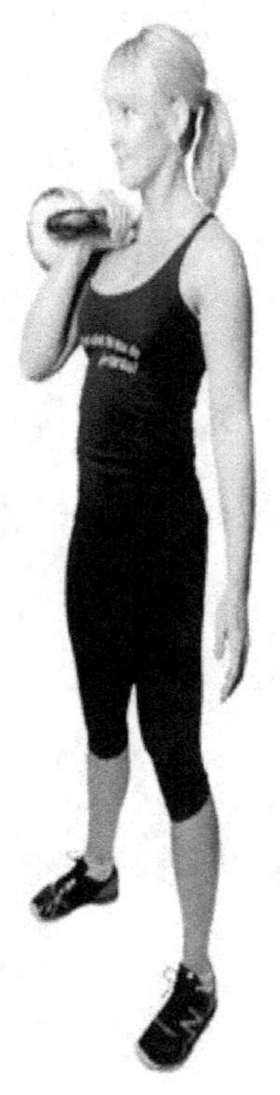

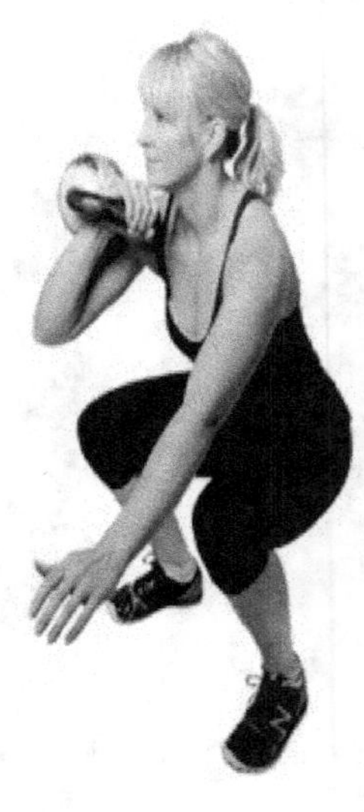

Next is _The Racked Reverse Lunge_. The _Rack Reverse Lunge_ works the lower back, shoulders, abdominals, calves, gluteus maximus, and hamstrings. This is one of the best moves you can do to work pretty much every single muscle in your legs. It requires great balance, and stability so it's great for your core.

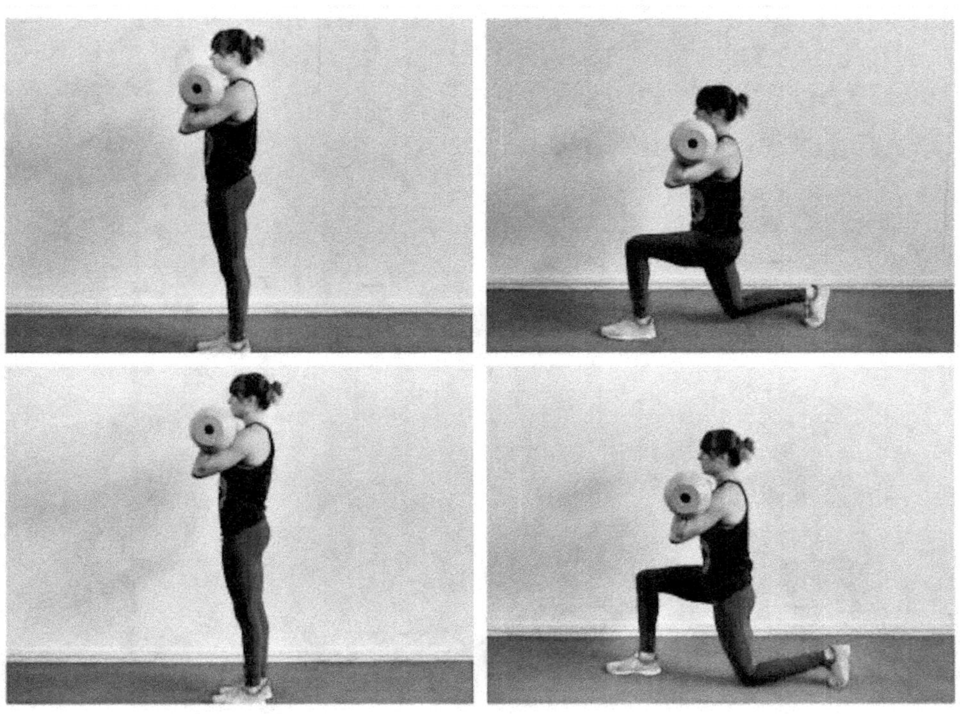

Next is _The Side Lunge & Clean_. _The Side Lunge & Clean_ is a incredibly effective move. Any advance kettlebell user will tell you that this move works wonders for most every aspect of your body. _The Side Lunge & Clean_ works the gluteus maximus, abductors, quads, hamstrings, soleus, tibias anterior, chest, shoulders, back, biceps, triceps, and abs. It's one of the most powerful compound movements in the Kettlebell world. 15 minutes of _The Side Lunge & Clean_ is considered an advanced kettlebell workout.

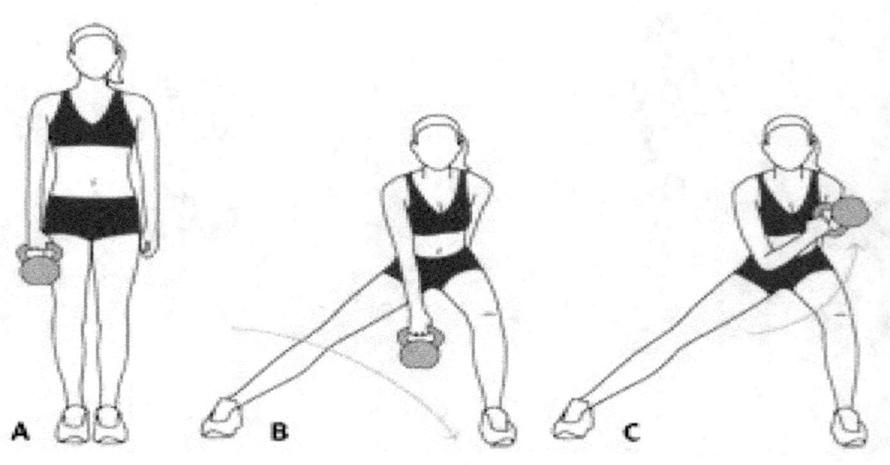

Next is *The One Leg Clean & Press*. This is a truly an advanced level move. When it comes to improving your balance, and stability no move is more effective. *The One Leg Clean & Press will push your balance to the limit. If you can do this without wobbling you have the balance of ah yoga master. Check it out here:* https://www.youtube.com/watch?v=vb-Aoow2zXc

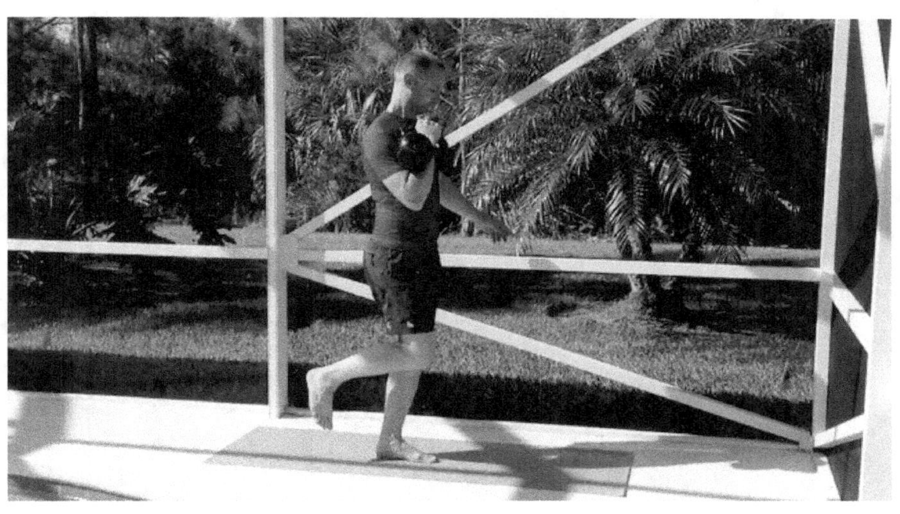

Next is *The Clean Squat Press*. *The Clean Squat Press* works the shoulders, traps, triceps middle lower back, abdominals, gluten, quadriceps, hamstrings, and calves. It's an interesting compound movement that works pretty much every major muscle group in the body.

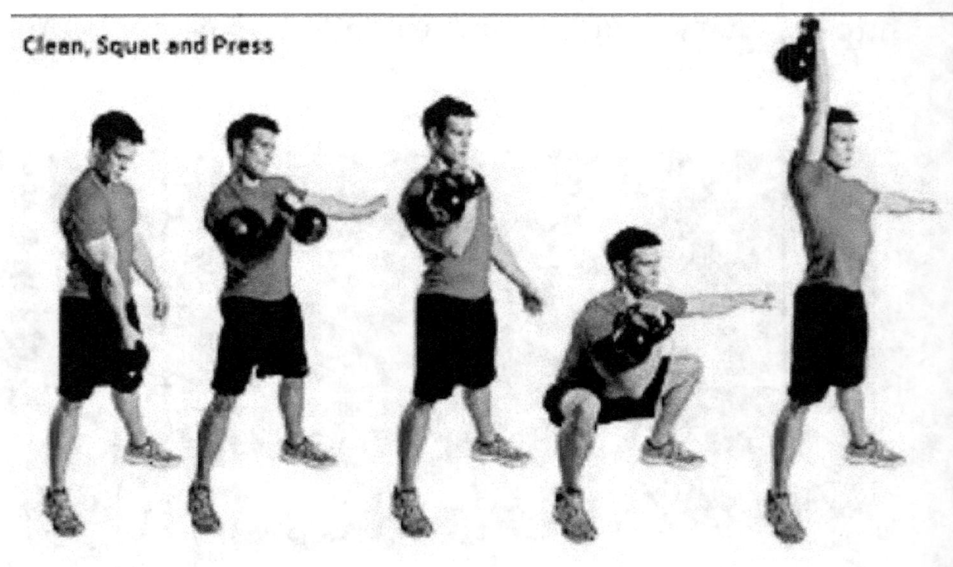

Next is _The Lateral Swing_. _The Lateral Swing_ is a complex movement that requires extreme control. If you think you're going to let go of the Kettlebell for one second than you need to stop. *The Lateral Swing* will cut body fat like a steak knife. If you combine *The Kettlebell Swing* with *The Changing Hand Swing,* and *The Lateral Swing* you got yourself a 30-minute workout that will have you ready for summer!

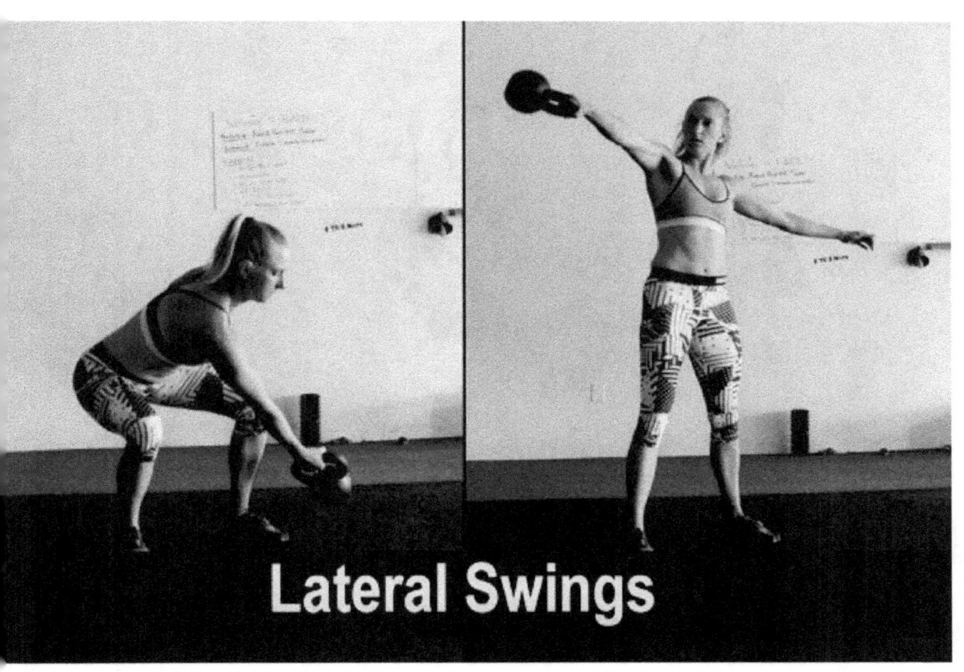

Last but not least is *The Pistol Squat*. I put *The Pistol Squat* last because to me it is the most difficult move. *The Pistol Squat* works the hips, hamstrings, quadriceps, gluteus maximus, and calves. It's the most effective workout to do when trying to strengthen individual legs. If you can't do *The Pistol Squat* without the Kettlebell don't try it with the Kettlebell.

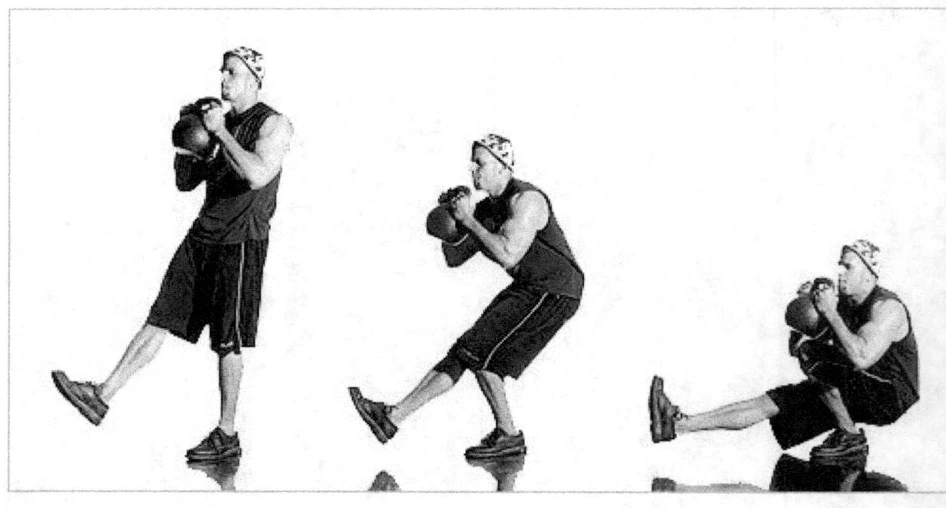

These advanced level workouts will have you ready for anything. The Kettlebell works out the entire body from head to toe building plenty of muscle endurance. You'll notice you have plenty of energy, stamina, and focus throughout the day. The Kettlebell is a time-tested tool. It's more ancient than any workout machine in any gym. To be exact the kettlebell is from the 1700s. An hour of any Kettlebell workout burns 1200 calories. There are 3500 calories in a pound so three hours of kettlebell burns a pound! How about that!

Motivation

All it takes is motivation. With motivation we all move forward. With motivation we overcome our weaknesses, and take control of our destinies. If there's anything in your life that has held you back allow the thought of you overcoming, and rising above it to motivate you. Allow the thought of better health to become a reality. With better health we all look at life differently. The more exercise that we offer our body the better our mind works. If we know what's negative in our life than we know what the sickness is. There are millions of people in this world that don't know what their problem is. They have no way of identifying the true issues that plagues their body. If you can look in the mirror, and stare your problem right in the face than you have something that they don't, and that's hope. You can hope for a better tomorrow because you can identify the problem. If you can identify the problem than you can find a solution. If your problem is lack of energy, strength, and coordination *The Kettlebell Cleanse* is the solution. If your problem is obesity *The Kettlebell Cleanse* is the solution. In this world very few people get to see the best version of themselves. Become the best version of you mentally, and physically, and watch the world around you change. When I became the best version of myself physically, and mentally, I became a different person. It's not all about the physical progression that you make. It's about the feeling the bell gives you. You will start to feel great in so many different ways. The way the bell made me feel was my guiding light. Every day I woke up happy, healthier, and cheerful. For once it felt like I did something to change my circumstances. At times I felt as if the hand dealt to me was permanent, and that there was nothing that I could do. After trying so many different avenues I begin to understand that weight loss is much more complex. Infomercials made it seem easy. Get this product, and you'll be ready for summer in a month. The truth is nothing like that exists. It's an unfortunate realization.

Body fat percentage is everything. Being a 200-pound man could mean anything depending on your body fat percentage. If your 6 foot 2 200 pounds 50% body fat that's not good! If your 6 foot 2 200 pounds 12% body fat that's amazing. The deciding factor is your body fat percentage. How much of your body is muscle, and how much of your body is fat. The more you tip the scale towards muscle the easier it is for you to lose fat, and keep it off. A lot of people talk about turning fat into muscle, but there is no such thing. If you're trying to gain muscle you eat more calories than your body requires while lifting weights. If you're trying to lose fat you eat less calories than your body requires while lifting weights. The problem is people use cardio equipment to try to lose weight. The issue with this is this type of exercise burns muscle, and fat indiscriminately. When using the treadmill you're not building muscle, but you are using energy. Your body is looking for a fuel source so that you can continue to run. It will get it from muscle, or fat. Compare that to a weighted cardio exercise. In this case you're actually using your muscles. So instead of you burning muscle, and fat you'll be preserving muscle, and burning fat. You want to lose weight without losing muscle.

Let's say you are a female, and your 5 foot 6 200 pounds 40% body fat. You lose 40 pounds doing cardio. Now you're 5 foot 6 160 pounds 50% body fat. That's still going to look bad. Body fat percentage is what's important not how much you weigh. If you lose that same 40 pounds with the Kettlebell your body fat percentage is going to go down. If you're 160 pounds, and you're 40% body fat 64 pounds of you is pure fat the rest is lean muscle. Now let's pretend that you lost this weight using the Kettlebell. You go from 200 to 160, but you've lost nothing, but pure body fat, and just a little muscle. This means your 160 pounds, and 25% body fat. That's going to look wonderful. You want to hold on to your muscle, and get rid of your fat. That's the key to genuine weight loss. You can make all of this happen if you stay motivated, and follow the program. Mix and match these exercises 5 days a week for 30 minutes to an hour. I guarantee you'll see, and feel the difference. You just have to stay motivated.

Vitamin Intake

Let me start this off by saying that by no means am I telling you to buy any of these vitamins. I'm just telling you the vitamins that I used during *The Kettlebell Cleanse*. I have no idea if they had an effect on my results, but I feel like they're worth mentioning. My vitamin intake during *The Kettlebell Cleanse* was well rounded. I tried to make sure I covered every single function of my body. Let's start things off with the first vitamin I took.

Ubiquinol is said to be very good for your cardiovascular health, and the last thing I wanted going out on me was my heart because I had high blood pressure. Ubiquinol was a supplement I took to make sure I had a little extra energy. Its supposed to be an incredibly powerful antioxidant it's also supposed to promote energy production as well, and I needed all the energy that I could get. They say it's good for brain health, and protecting the cells from free radicals. To be honest I still use ubiquinol it's much better than

Co q-10 because it's easily absorb into the body.

The second thing I kind of supplemented with was *Apple Cider Vinegar With Mother*. I mixed my apple cider vinegar with a teaspoon of lemon juice, eight ounces of water, and made sure to take this every single day at least 2 times a day. I have no idea what kind of effect it may have had on my progression. I just know that it's still apart of my routine to this day. Apple cider vinegar is supposed to promote weight loss. I have no idea if it contributed to my weight loss, but I feel like it's worth mentioning.

The third supplement that I used was *Black Seed Oil*. Black seed oil is supposed to be the God of all supplements. It's supposed to promote health across the board. They say that it's a huge anti-inflammatory. Since pretty much every health problem is caused by inflammation black seed oil is probably the number one vitamin you can use. They say black seed oil is wonderful for cancer prevention and treatment. They also say it's crucial to liver health. They say that it prevents diabetes. They also say it's great for weight loss which was one of the main reasons why I started using it. They say that it's great for your hair, nails, and skin. They also say that it's wonderful for fighting off infections, and that it's effective against certain strains of superbugs that most antibiotics are not working on anymore. Black seed oil has been studied over, and over again. It's probably one of the most studied supplements on the market so there's some solid science to back up what it does. Still I have no idea if it had a major effect on my workout or not nor do I have any idea if it helped my weight loss.

Another supplement I used was *Grapeseed, Green Tea, & Pine Bark Complex*. The combination of these creates a super antioxidant. The main reason why I was taking it was for energy. The combination of these three things promotes a natural boost in energy. It's not like a caffeine pill or anything like that it's something that works overtime. This is one of those supplements that I don't like running out of I try to make sure that I keep it in stock as much as I possibly can.

I used _Probiotics_ because they support your immune system. They're supposed to introduce positive bacteria back into your stomach. This is supposed to help your digestive system, and promote weight loss. I can say that I got sick a lot less often once I start taking the probiotics. Still I started sprinting around the same time so I can't really say which one was super effective.

L-Carnitine was one of the first supplements that I started using. It aids in transforming fat into energy. This is the most important process in weight loss, and energy production. Also it's supposed to aid in muscle building as well. It's supposed to be one of the main elements of muscle building. A lot of bodybuilders use L-Carnitine, and some even say it helps with your overall brain health. Now I don't know if it did any of these things for me I just know during _The Kettlebell Cleanse_ I took it everyday.

Omega-3 Fish Oil is something that I've been taking since I was a kid. It's supposed to support cardiovascular health, and cognitive function. It supports your immune system, your bone health, and your joint health as well. It's also said to support a healthy mood. I don't know if it does any of these things I just know that my mom has been giving me omega-3 fish oil since I was a kid. It's supposed to be one of the most important vitamins on the planet for preserving your body, and promoting overall health.

Vitamin D3 is a supplement I started taking when I realize that I probably wasn't getting enough of it. Vitamin D comes from sun exposure, and since I don't really go outside too often I knew that I probably was vitamin D3 deficient. Vitamin D3 is supposed to support bone destiny, the immune system, and boost absorption of calcium. It's supposed to support neuromuscular function whatever that means. All I know is Vitamin D3 is very important to the body, and if you're not getting enough sunlight than most likely you're not getting enough vitamin D3. Still I have no idea if it had any effect on my performance whatsoever.

Biotin is something that I also supplemented with. It's supposed to be good for your hair, nails, and skin. It's also supposed to support some other viable functions in the body. I guess biotin is one of the key ingredients that your hair needs to grow. That's one of the main reasons why I was supplementing with it. I will say when I started to use it I did notice a difference in my hair quality, nail quality, and the appearance of my skin. It took about three to four months though. Still I'm not sure if that was the sprinting or the biotin or a combination of both.

    Sea kelp was something else that I used. It's supposed to be a source of iodine. Iodine is important for thyroid function. The thyroid regulates a huge amount of functions in your body including your hormonal balance. Your hormonal balance has a huge effect on your energy levels, your mood, and also your weight. If your thyroid isn't functioning properly than most likely you're going to have weight issues. They say this is why the Japanese are so skinny because their diet is rich in iodine. It's because they eat so much seaweed. Still I have no idea if it had any effect on my weight loss.

Garcinia Cambogia is supposed to stop your body from creating new fat. It was featured on Dr. Oz a while ago, and it's supposed to be proven to actually stop your body from creating new fat. Now I'm not sure if it stopped my body from creating new fat all I know is that it was a part of my everyday regimen.

Of course I took a _Multi Vitamin_ because that just makes common sense. Everybody probably takes a multi-vitamin I've been taking one since I was a kid. It's always been apart of my regimen.

African Mango was also something that I included in my supplement regimen. It's supposed to help promote weight loss but there isn't much research behind it to say that it does anything of any kind of significance. Still a lot of people swear by it so I added it to my supplement pile.

I also took _L-Theanine_, and if you're a coffee drinker like me L-Theanine is absolutely essential. It gets rid of that jittery affect that coffee gives you, and makes it a smooth high. It also has some other benefits that might be worth mentioning. Apparently in 1964 Japan approved L-Theanine for unlimited use in all foods. L-Theanine has been linked to relieving stress. It's the key ingredient in green tea, which has been linked to relieving stress.

I'm not endorsing any of these vitamins in anyway. I'm just informing you of the supplements I used during *The Kettlebell Cleanse*. These supplements may have enhanced my results, and it wouldn't be fair if I didn't mention them. If you choose to take them my best advice is to have a conversation with your doctor. If you want to know the exact supplements that I used than check out my website http://workoutkingrule.blogspot.com/.

Mind Your Diet

If you don't pay attention to what you eat you're not going to be able to accomplish anything. In this situation I'm speaking about eating for energy not eating for weight loss. Remember *The Kettlebell Cleanse* takes a lot of energy. If you're not eating for energy than you're not going to be able to last for very long. Your body is going to need power so therefore you have to eat the foods that give you the most power. I'm going to give you a detailed example of the type of foods I ate during *The Kettlebell Cleanse*. You can either mimic this, or find similar foods that might give you the drive you need.

First thing in the morning I made sure to blend a shake. I blended kale, oranges, apples, bananas, blueberries, cranberries, strawberries, and I used apple juice instead of water. I did research on each one of these fruits, and vegetables to make sure that they would give me the optimum performance that I was seeking.

Kale is the healthiest vegetable you can eat. I made sure to put more kale in my shake than anything else. Every single fruit that I mention I used a whole one. I used a whole orange, a whole apple, and ah whole banana. I used about maybe eight cranberries, eight blueberries, and about four strawberries. To be honest after I took the shake in the morning I always would feel wonderful. It was probably the best part of my diet, and a great way to kick off my day. I also had oatmeal because I wanted to make sure that I was getting an extreme amount of fiber.

The combination of these fruits and vegetables gave me an extreme amount of energy. It's probably the one thing that I can attest to my newfound power. It actually boosts my energy level. I don't know if any of my vitamins did anything to actually boost my energy level, but I'm sure my shake did the job. To be honest over time it became even more effective. Most people don't understand that eating healthy is something that takes time to affect your body. Sometimes you'll be able to feel it right away, but a lot of people quit because they don't feel any difference within a few days, or a week. I noticed after a month of taking the shake my overall mood in general changed. Remember I told you I was a very tired, cranky, and moody individual. I was so overweight my body had absolutely no energy whatsoever. When your body has no energy it pretty much ruins everything. You don't want to do anything. I can say that this shake had a profound effect on that mindset, and was a key ingredient in making *The Kettlebell Cleanse* much more effective. I made sure that I didn't add any sugar to the mix. I also made sure to put cinnamon in my oatmeal. The cinnamon had a profound effect on my health as well. Remember cinnamon is nothing but pure fiber, and fiber is incredibly important to the digestive system. As long as you're going to the bathroom often you're losing weight. You want to make sure you're getting as much fiber as you possibly can. That's why I added apples to the mix because apples are rich in fiber. It's also why I added blueberries to the mix because they're rich in fiber as well. I wanted to make sure that I upped my fiber intake by as much as I possibly could. I also wanted to make sure I was getting a ton of vitamin C.

Vitamin C is the reason why I made sure to add a whole orange. I added bananas to the mix because I wanted to make sure that I was getting a lot of potassium. Bananas are good for Vitamin B6. Vitamin B6 is something that you'll see in almost every natural energy supplement.

Cranberries were just another source of fiber. They have even more fiber than blueberries. They're also packed full of antioxidants. The strawberries were mostly for flavor at first until I started doing more research, and I realize that strawberries were amazing. They can help prevent heart disease, stroke, cancer, high blood pressure, constipation, allergies, asthma diabetes, and depression. Strawberries are ah incredibly effective antioxidant.

Oatmeal is packed full of iron it's probably one of the most iron rich foods out there. It also has an extremely large amount of vitamin B6, magnesium, and vitamin A not to mention 6 grams of protein. Speaking of protein maybe I should discuss what I had for lunch.

Everyday for lunch I would have grilled chicken, beans, and a protein shake. My lunch was all about protein intake. For lunch I wanted to make sure I was getting as much protein in my body as possible. That's why I made sure I had grilled chicken because chicken has an extremely large amount of protein. Chicken is one of the most protein rich meats on the planet, and it's healthier for you than beef or pork. Not to mention it's a lot easier to cook especially if you know how to bake. It's even easier if you have a griller like one of those commercial grillers that drain out all the grease. Everyday when I woke up in the morning I would turn on my rice cooker, and add one cup or two cups of black beans. I chose black beans because they're low in calories. One cup is only 624 calories, and because they are extremely high in dietary fiber, you get 29 grams in one cup. Also because they're high in protein you get 39 grams of protein in one cup. They have an extremely large amount of iron, and ah extremely large amount of magnesium, and calcium so it was an obvious choice. Black beans are ah incredibly healthy super food with 2760 mg of potassium.

The body is supposed to consume at least 30 to 38 grams of fiber every day if you're a man. If you're a woman it's about 25 grams of fiber everyday. So basically one cup of black beans would almost be enough fiber for the day for a man and more than enough for a woman. If you read up on black beans you'll understand just how nutritious they really are. It's one of the most underestimated super foods on the planet. The only substitute that I would ever use for black beans if I didn't have them is quinoa. Quinoa is probably the greatest food on the planet, and the only food that has pretty much all the amino acids that you need. I also made sure that I had a whey protein isolate shake everyday.

For dinner I ate pretty much anything I wanted. I just made sure that I didn't eat any fast food. I completely cut out fast food in general. For dinner I would have a meal with black beans on the side. I would have ground turkey meat, chicken, or fish. I wouldn't have any beef or pork. So I would have some turkey tacos with black beans, and cheese, or I would have some turkey nachos with black beans, and cheese. Sometimes I would eat some salmon, beans, and rice. As long as I added the black beans to the meal I would create any combination I wanted. Eating beans with your meal helps the digestive process. It increases the nutritional value of the meal. I didn't really eat any dessert, but I've never been one to eat dessert anyway so it wasn't a big change for me.

My diet wasn't too extreme it wasn't anything that was impractical. All my food was good it wasn't like I had to eat nasty stuff that I didn't like. When you have to eat a bunch of nasty stuff that you don't like eventually you're going to give up on it. I loved the food I was eating! My shake was delicious, and my oatmeal was always good especially with cinnamon. I never put sugar in my oatmeal I just added cinnamon to it. If I wanted it to taste good I would add some honey. I made sure that I got my honey from the whole food store. Black beans are my favorite especially once you season them with some Lawry's, and some pepper. The grilled chicken was always good because I mean grilled chicken is awesome. Sometimes I would grill chicken and have a chicken black bean salad. It tasted great! My diet gave me energy, power, and change my mood all together. It's the main reason why I was able to go on. If I never changed my diet I would have never saw any positive effects from *The Kettlebell Cleanse* in the first place because I wouldn't be able to do it. My intention was never to change my diet for weight loss, but to promote energy production. I simply wanted to feel better, and run longer, and this diet accomplished that for me. I didn't find it difficult. If you can find food that has similar nutritious value that you actually find delicious by all means go about it in your own way. I'm just telling you exactly what I did. I don't want to leave any details out because that might be the one detail that contributed to my progression. If you choose to follow my diet to the letter it is more likely that you will see the same results that I did. Maybe you might find some loopholes that I didn't find. You might be able to improve upon the diet. If so please don't hoard information comment, and add your perspective. Tell the people of the dietary changes you implement that worked in combination with _The Kettlebell Cleanse._ Maybe tells us some of the vitamins that you used in combination with _The Kettlebell Cleanse_. Share other forms of kettlebell training you've tried in combination with _The Kettlebell Cleanse_ that worked for you.

Wrap Up

The Kettlebell community is becoming more popular. There's a lot of misinformation out there. I put this book out so some competent information would be available. When you go online, and look at some of the forms none of the messaging is correct. It's all rather vague, and sometimes over-inflated. Can you expect real results with the Kettle bell? Of course! Just don't expect these over-inflated results that you've been hearing about online. It's true that the kettlebell burns 1200 calories an hour. This means you can burn a pound of fat in 3 days if you do an hour everyday. That is an undeniable benefit of the Kettlebell. The problem is people don't tell you that you have to up the weight. They also don't include all these different variations of exercise. The Kettlebell is a core concentrated tool. With a powerful core you can use the Kettlebell in a number of ways. As long as you're willing to put in the effort you'll gain results. If you're trying to lose weight pick a kettlebell that's the right size for you. If you're trying to gain muscle than you need a kettlebell that weighs more. In my opinion if you have a friend, or a partner to do this kind of exercise with it really makes it easy. Every single day me, and my girlfriend who is now my wife would workout with kettlebells. Doing this together really helped us both stay focus. Try to partner up with one person or even a group of people it really makes it easier. Stick to the diet it will increase your energy. Stay consistent, and enjoy yourself. With that I bid you farewell. I'm the Workout King have a great life, and great health.